Michael,

Even though the last time we spoke was one year ago... I hope you are taking an interest in your financial affairs. Possibly this book will help.

Please enjoy,

Brian

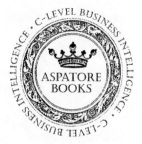

www.Aspatore.com

Aspatore Books is the largest and most exclusive publisher of C-Level executives (CEO, CFO, CTO, CMO, Partner) from the world's most respected companies and law firms. Aspatore annually publishes a select group of C-Level executives from the Global 1,000, top 250 law firms (Partners & Chairs), and other leading companies of all sizes. C-Level Business Intelligence™, as conceptualized and developed by Aspatore Books, provides professionals of all levels with proven business intelligence from industry insiders – direct and unfiltered insight from those who know it best – as opposed to third-party accounts offered by unknown authors and analysts. Aspatore Books is committed to publishing an innovative line of business and legal books, those which lay forth principles and offer insights that when employed, can have a direct financial impact on the reader's business objectives, whatever they may be. In essence, Aspatore publishes critical tools – need-to-read as opposed to nice-to-read books – for all business professionals.

Inside the Minds

The critically acclaimed *Inside the Minds* series provides readers of all levels with proven business intelligence from C-Level executives (CEO, CFO, CTO, CMO, Partner) from the world's most respected companies. Each chapter is comparable to a white paper or essay and is a future-oriented look at where an industry/profession/topic is heading and the most important issues for future success. Each author has been carefully chosen through an exhaustive selection process by the *Inside the Minds* editorial board to write a chapter for this book. *Inside the Minds* was conceived in order to give readers actual insights into the leading minds of business executives worldwide. Because so few books or other publications are actually written by executives in industry, *Inside the Minds* presents an unprecedented look at various industries and professions never before available.

INSIDE THE MINDS

Inside the Minds:
Wealth Strategies for Doctors

*Leading Financial Planners on Investing Techniques for Building &
Maintaining Wealth*

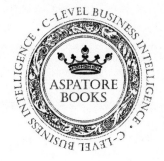

Published by Aspatore, Inc.

For corrections, company/title updates, comments or any other inquiries please email info@aspatore.com.

First Printing, 2004
10 9 8 7 6 5 4 3 2 1

ISBN 158762060X

Inside the Minds Managing Editor, Carolyn Murphy; Edited by Emily High; Cover design by Scott Rattray & Ian Mazie

Inside the Minds:
Wealth Strategies for Doctors

*Leading Financial Planners on Investing Techniques for Building &
Maintaining Wealth*

CONTENTS

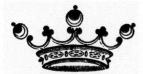

A Primer for Holistic Financial Health

Brian Grodman

Founder
Grodman Financial Group

The 21st Century Doctor

Doctors graduate from medical school with an enormous debt load; at times these debts exceed $200,000. The starting compensation for physicians is usually around $100,000-$150,000 annually, which makes paying back this debt quite difficult. Furthermore, hospitals and their affiliates now own many physicians' practices, reducing the potential for tax write-offs and overall compensation. The doctor of the 21st century is more likely to be an employee, as opposed to the 20th century independent physician. This generally contributes to case overload, lack of freedom, and bureaucracy. All of these additional pressures can be a source of great frustration, over and beyond the usual financial woes.

The Early Focus

To begin designing a wealth strategy for a client in the medical profession, we need to first list all assets, liabilities and cash flow. We can then determine how best to utilize the cash flow to maximize net worth (assets – liabilities). A simple spreadsheet should be constructed twice each year to monitor progress. From this starting point, the doctor and financial planner can work together to counteract the stresses and frustrations of the 21st century doctor.

The early years of employment should be devoted to reducing "bad" debt. This is either non-deductible loans (i.e. auto, school, credit cards, etc.) or deductible high interest debt. Once this has been accomplished, pre-tax retirement contributions should be maximized in almost all cases. Doctors without children should not obtain large life insurance policies. Instead, they should place any extra funds in growth-oriented investments.

Physicians with dependents should obtain guaranteed 20-30 year term life insurance that has the option for conversion

Most doctors should not be concerned with choosing individual stocks or mutual funds. The focus should be on building an all-around portfolio that mirrors their risk tolerance. They should make sure they can sleep at night, given the balance of the portfolio. A mixture of investments should have the effect of lowering volatility without hampering potential return.

If possible, the doctor should purchase the office in which he or she works. The doctor will then have more control over his work situation. Real estate rarely reduces in value. The doctor should always have 3-6 months in fairly liquid investments should a financial emergency occur.

Investment Specialists

The doctor should spend very little time managing investments. By using a trusted financial planner, the doctor can minimize the concerns of micromanaging the portfolio. The general population utilizes the service of a physician due to his or her specialty. Likewise, the doctor should utilize a financial professional with whom he or she is comfortable due to the planner's financial specialty.

The financial plan should then be monitored semi-annually, barring any special circumstances. The strategy should also be updated when any major life event occurs (such as marriage, divorce, birth of a child, inheritance, job change, retirement, etc.). The "financial plan" does not have to be in the form of a thick book. It may simply be a dozen or fewer action items.

A skilled financial planner can help the doctor realize that the goal of the wealth strategy should mirror the life goals of the investor. The rate of return should *never* be the goal. The realization of desires and aspirations is always the goal. The money earned is simply how these goals can be accomplished.

Preparing to Plan

Often it is helpful to ask yourself a number of questions before deciding on and implementing a wealth strategy with a financial planner. To ensure that nothing is forgotten in this critical meeting, be sure to know your response to each of the following questions:

➤ How much do I expect to pay for my children's education?

➤ When do I want to retire?

➤ Do I plan to earn money after I retire?

➤ How much do I want to work during the next five years, and how will this impact my earnings?

➤ How much of a monthly or annual portfolio decline can I stomach (5%, 10%, etc)?

➤ What are my current cash flow needs? Will they change during retirement?

➤ Do I really enjoy my profession? If not, will I want to change careers or specialty?

> ➢ How do I want my estate distributed? In what time frame?

> ➢ Who should be my executor, trustee and guardian listed in my estate plan?

A Formulaic Approach

For doctors who are seeking to find a comprehensive and efficient financial plan for their goals, I have found this outline to be a very helpful guide throughout the process:

A.   First, make an asset/liability spreadsheet as previously described. An Excel-type spreadsheet should list the assets on the top (by ownership) and liabilities towards the bottom. An example of a typical asset/liability spreadsheet can be found in Appendix A. This spreadsheet should be updated twice per year using the following column on the right. A determination can then be made regarding the success of the plan.

B.   Monitor the spreadsheet semi-annually.

C.   Pay off "bad" debt, as described earlier in the chapter.

D.   Start a tax-deferred savings program. The employer will usually set up this program. The maximum contribution is usually appropriate, with the investments going into growth funds.

E.   Coordinate the plan with your financial advisor, accountant, and attorney. Too often, the lack of coordination causes a major problem down the road. This could relate to business entity structure, beneficiary designation, ownership, or a myriad of other issues.

F.   Make sure beneficiaries and contingent beneficiaries are listed on appropriate documents. These documents include annuities, IRA's, life insurance and retirement plans.

G.   Benchmark investment returns annually. An appropriate benchmark should be decided initially. This will prevent second-guessing at the end of the time period.

H.   Do not micromanage investments. Whether the investor manages the portfolio with assistance, or alone, do not check on performance more than monthly. This only causes needless angst and ulcers. Looking at the account often does not cause it to increase in value!

All of these steps should occur within a three-month period. Often, a certain degree of momentum is needed to accomplish many of these mundane tasks. Of course, the monitoring should be done periodically for the duration of the investor's lifetime.

A Savings Case Study

If a certain investor wanted to accumulate $1 million in thirty years and started with nothing – he or she would need to contribute $1,000 each month, assuming a 6% return. However, this example excludes the impact of taxes. If the tax rate on all growth was 16%, then the *net* annual return of 5% would mandate increasing the monthly cash flow to $1,200. Thus, a 16% reduction in growth necessitates a 20% funding increase. This common example leaves out one important factor. Once the $1 million goal has been achieved, the after tax dollars (5% money in our example) can be withdrawn tax-free. Conversely, the pretax money (6%) must be taxed upon withdrawal during retirement. Overall, it is always important to prioritize funding for retirement above educating children. There are loans available for funding college, but not for funding retirement.

What to Expect

Many misguided individuals take the wrong approach in their efforts to profit in the market. We believe in assuming a more balanced perspective in terms of the stock matrket. In our view, if we can simply match the appropriate benchmark while reducing volatility, we have succeeded. The benchmark may be the Standard & Poor's 500™, the Morgan Stanley World Index™, or a combination of many indexes.

Managing money should be done with the brain, not the heart. The financial plan should be maintained during both up and down markets, since it has nothing to do with market performance. It's important to expect downturns and not let them affect your previously established plan.

In the next five years, I believe that doctors can also expect the cost of investing (market friction) will continue to decrease. This has happened to some degree already with the decimalization of the stock market. In the coming years, additional pressures will be placed on the mutual fund industry to reduce fees as well.

Brian Grodman is a Certified Financial Planner™ practitioner specializing in Investment Management, Tax Reduction Strategies, Retirement Planning, Insurance Consulting and Estate Planning. His financial planning career began in 1985.

Mr. Grodman holds a Bachelor of Science degree from the University of Massachusetts - Amherst, where he pursued an engineering core curriculum, and an MBA degree from Babson College. He holds the Certified Financial Plannner (CFP)® designation from the College for Financial Planning and the Certified Fund Specialist (CFS) designation from the Institute of Certified Fund Specialists. In addition, he was one of only 800 financial planners admitted to the prestigious Registry of the International Association for Financial Planning (IAFP).

Grodman Financial Group, LLC is a Registered Investment Advisor with the State of New Hampshire Bureau of Securities Regulation. Brian is a Registered Principal with Jefferson Pilot Securities Corporation. He holds the Chartered Financial Consultant (ChFC) and Chartered Life Underwriter (CLU) designations from the American College.

Brian supervised and trained over 1200 investment professionals for one of the largest financial services companies in the United States, Chubb LifeAmerica. In 1995, Mr. Grodman was elected to the 12-member General Agents Advisory Committee (GAAC). This respected committee served in an advisory capacity on behalf of 1500 financial services professionals within Jefferson Pilot Financial. He served as chairman of its Securities Committee from 1996-1999. Brian was the youngest president to serve the GAAC, being elected for the fiscal year 1998-1999.

From 1992 through 1997 he served as president of the International Association for Financial Planning-New Hampshire/Vermont chapter. The October 1996, 1997 and September 1998 issues of <u>Worth Magazine</u> along with the July 1998, November 1999, August 2000, and December 2002 issues of <u>Medical Economics</u> listed Brian as one of the "Best Financial Advisors in the United States."* His many articles and comments have been published and/or quoted by a variety of magazines, trade publications and newspapers including Medical Economics, The Boston Globe, The New York Times, The Manchester Union Leader, Business NH Magazine, and New Hampshire Editions. He has lectured at financial planning seminars across the country and on the open seas.

*Information regarding either survey is available upon request.

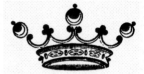

Financial Planning Basics: A *Must* for Doctors

M. Eileen Dorsey

President
Money Consultants Advisory, Inc.

Realistic Grounding for Medical Professionals

As a Certified Financial Planner Practitioner, I feel that my job is to help people balance what they need with what they want. My philosophy is to combine my technical expertise with the reality of what people need, what they want and how the world really works. What works in theory does not necessarily work in the real world because people do not always do what they are supposed to do and the world does not work the way we want it to.

In the real world, most people are somewhat nervous about principal volatility even if they tell you they won't be, people focus on the short-term rather than the long-term even though we advise them not to, human beings have emergencies, and our product marketing gurus convince people to buy now and pay later. In my experience with clients in the medical profession, I have found that doctors tend to be more aggressive than they really are.

Doctors tend to be more aggressive investors than the average person because of their confidence and success. Confident and successful people tend to be willing to take more risk than the average smart, but less confident and less successful person. Part of this is due to the confidence in their earnings ability. However, doctors are also well educated and realistic enough to understand some of the principles of risk – primarily that you have to take high risk to get high return and that just because you take high risk does not guarantee high return. They are willing to accept education about the investment process as it relates to risk, reward and asset allocation. They are also educated enough to stay focused on their goals (e.g. accumulating a large enough nest egg to build a retirement portfolio to provide sufficient income in retirement).

I do not think that we as advisers are responsible if the client does not do what he or she is supposed to do as outlined and agreed upon in the "plan," but I want to do the best job I can for the people that I advise and because of this I try to take into consideration all the "what ifs." This gives my clients a better chance to achieve their financial goals. And that is always the bottom line.

A good plan is one that works for the client and helps them achieve their financial goals. Typically this type of plan would follow generally accepted financial planning guidelines customized to the comfort level of the client, where they are in life, and their specific financial objectives and accompanying time frame. The operative word is *customized,* which means it is personalized and not boiler plate. Their goals, of course, must be realistic and achievable. Their expectations must also be realistic.

Financial Plan Maintenance

After a doctor's specific goals and needs have been intricately analyzed and a tailored plan has been created, the plan must then be implemented. Implementation and maintenance are essential steps that can often break the line in what is otherwise a sturdy financial plan. The plan must be reviewed and revised as the variables in the clients' lives change, and these variables change frequently for everyone.

Their income may change. They may get married, divorced, have children or additional children. Their practice may change. They may go from employer or partner status to employee status or vice versa. Their needs for insurance such as life, disability or health may change. The asset allocation may change because one of the asset classes has grown faster than the others. Their risk tolerance may change simply because they are getting older and closer to retirement or because the extended bear market scared them. As they change employment status their benefits change. The plan should thus be under a constant monitoring process, or at the very minimum, on an annual basis. Also, assumptions about inflation and rates of return need to be changed periodically.

Long-Term Relationships

I do not consider myself an investment guru. I simply consider myself an adviser that utilizes the financial planning process in working with clients. The financial planning process forces us to do things the right way, in a very structured relationship. I believe that the most important part of the investment process is determining "real" comfort level or as the industry calls it, the investment philosophy. I also need to figure out what clients will *actually* do, rather than what they say they will do. This understanding is best achieved in a long-term relationship. The more intimately I know a person, the better the job that I will be able to do for them. Additionally, the longer I know the individual, the better the job that I can do for them. Long-term relationships become extremely important in this business. Also, if we develop this kind of long-term relationship I can be right there on the same page with the client and already familiar with their situation when (not if) he or she has a financial crisis. This is oftentimes more of an intangible benefit which is not actually realized or appreciated until that time of dire need. Even though most doctors are focused more on specific investments and not on financial planning, I still feel that I must get to know the total person in order to do a good job for them and that with financial planning I can also provide a much better investment experience.

Stick to the Basics to Benefit

My personal philosophy is that most people spend their entire lives searching for the perfect investment rather than maximizing the amount going into their plan and directing this into good basic investments. For most people wealth accumulation has more to do with how much they save and avoiding large losses and bad investments, and only a little to do with incremental performance of one good fund versus another good fund. I believe that the return *of* your principal is more important than the return *on* your principal. Unfortunately, it is simply the case that losses have a greater impact on long-term performance than gains. So the best way to win the investment game is to minimize the losses.

A perfect example is putting all of your eggs in one basket (such as growth stocks), as one such new client had done right before he came to see me. The money in his profit sharing plan was transferred to a high-performing growth stock fund at the peak of the growth stock market in 1999 and then transferred to bonds at the bottom of the growth stock market and close to the peak for bonds. Thus, rather than being constantly on the prowl for a new approach, a client should focus on maximizing the current plan.

Enabling Doctors to Tailor their Own Plan

In customizing a plan for my clients in the medical profession, I like to use payroll deduction, automatic savings plans and dollar-cost-averaging as much as possible because this helps ease the comfort level problem and the "procrastination problem." Most doctors are too busy to make the constant investment decisions that are necessary for a healthy plan. I do not think that I would be saving very much myself if I couldn't have the money automatically deducted. In a majority of cases, doctors simply do not have the time to sit down and write those checks. And each check writing session would involve another investment decision. The questions would be constantly echoing: Should I or shouldn't I? Is this still the best place to put my money?

Additionally, taxes have to be considered in the investment process; however, although almost half of our paycheck gets lost to taxes, it should not dominate the doctor's investment decision. I like to diversify tax strategies to the fullest extent possible. I think it's a wise plan to keep some in taxable for liquidity purposes and then pay as you go on the taxes. This offers more choices of how to take income during retirement, placing some in tax-free to ease the tax burden now *and* in the future. It would be great to keep everything in "real" tax-free but we do not have that option. For most doctors, the majority of their wealth outside of their home and their practice will thus end up in tax-deferred because of the 401(k), pensions, 403(b), IRAs, etc. but I do not want everything to end up there because of the lack of choice of taking retirement income and lack of liquidity and so on. These specific considerations can help the client to customize their plan to fit their lifestyle.

Laying the Foundations for a Doctor-Oriented Action Plan

The first step in developing a specific action plan is of course to meet with the doctor and their spouse and allow them get to know me and me to become acquainted with them. At this first meeting, I am then able to take in both their personal and financial history.

Also, a part of their specific plan and ongoing service includes helping them manage their practice. Even if the doctor is in fact an employee, we have to treat the practice as a business and help them manage it, which typically includes negotiating contracts and reviewing contracts, benefits and overhead alloation. This also involves their attorney. If they are solo practitioners and/or partners, this practice consulting on a personal level becomes more intense. This is a small part of the initial plan and a large part of the ongoing service.

In order to establish a strong sense of understanding between both parties at the first meeting with the doctor client, there are a number of critical items to discuss:

> Discuss client's goals and objectives and find out what they want to accomplish financially. A general estimate of the time frame in which they want to accomplish these goals is another integral piece of information to obtain. This will help present a better picture of exactly what your role will be as an adviser and what the client's expectations will be at each step along the way.

> Discuss the client's current financial profile and carefully review all financial information with them. I ask them to bring all documents such as current investment statements, paycheck stubs, prior tax returns, all insurance policies, employer-based benefits, estate planning documents, information about their practices, etc. It is amazing what tax returns (including backup data), credit card summary and canceled checks reveal about a person's money habits and lifestyle.

> Determine the client's comfort level by talking to them, discussing differences between fixed-guaranteed investments and the principal fluctuation of variable investments, discussing their current investments with them, the performance of these investments and how they fit their comfort level and financial objectives. It is important to talk to the client realistically about performance

expectations both current and past. Finding out about their prior investment experiences – what went wrong and what went right – can be crucial in developing a better investment strategy for them in the future.

> Help the client to develop a personal investment philosophy or select investment philosophy from samples and/or work through a risk tolerance test. Essentially this boils down to determining how much will be invested in safe guaranteed, how much in solid variable such as balanced, growth and income, blue-chip or large-cap stock funds and how much in more aggressive investments. Having the client think through whether he should buy and hold very consistent performers, passively rebalance asset classes, actively monitor or a combination of these strategies is the core purpose of these tests.

Discussing all of the above considerations lays the foreground for all of the interactions that will follow and therefore, the initial meeting is critical. Having this sort of in-depth discussion can take anywhere from one to six hours with the client, but it is essential to budget enough time to treat all of these issues.

After the First Meeting

Get to know client on paper. Examining a client's financial data without the client present will undoubtedly allow for a more in-depth review of the whole picture. This process can take anywhere in the range of ten to twenty hours.

> Analyze the client's current investments in conjunction with published information such as Morningstar.

➢ Determine the cost of short-term, intermediate-term and long-term goals and the time frame of each goal and translate this to their "monthly equivalent savings number," or how much they need to save on a monthly basis to achieve each goal. For example, for retirement funding I figure out how much they need to save on a monthly basis to retire at a specific retirement age and maintain their same standard of living until they die. The time frame is from now until estimated death. This is based on what they have accumulated to date, including money saved for them by others, such as their employer-paid pension and social security, and then subtract what they are saving or what their employer is saving for them. That gives me a net of any additional that they need to save. Another example of a targeted savings plan would be examining how much the client will need to save to send their 4 year-old to a private college or university whose tuition is currently $30,000 per year, assuming they want to fund 100%.

➢ Figure out how much long-term investing they can force into their spending plan. Get them to save to the "ouch point" – I've found this to be where it hurts a little but they can still afford it. Then, prorate as necessary depending on how much they can save and depending on the priority they have set in their goals.

➢ Develop starting point model asset allocation for the client. Determine what asset classes the client should be in.

➢ Reanalyze the client's current investments in terms of their comfort level and investment philosophy, where they are in life and their goals and objectives and recommended asset allocation and published information about the investment such as Morningstar data. Look at relative performance and most importantly *consistent* performance, beta, alpha, standard deviation, tenure of manager, R squared, turnover, equity and/or fixed income style such as value or growth, look for reasonable expense ratios, knowledge about the fund family, knowledge about how this fund/fund family works for current clients, etc.

➢ When determining specific asset allocation, make sure to include all investments including their 401(k), 403(b), profit sharing money, pension, value realistic value of practice, spouse's pension, etc. Do not make any isolated investment decisions. Look at the total picture.

➢ Prioritize the client's investment structure. Usually max before-tax savings plans such as pension and/or 401(k) or 403(b) first. Take advantage of payroll deduction and bank drafts into mutual funds and annuities. Don't forget about IRAs and college savings plans.

➢ Assign a hold or sell to their current investments.

➢ Develop repositioning recommendations as applicable and recommendations for future investments. I would rather error on the conservative side, but not so conservative that they do not get any growth. I would also rather error on the side of liquidity because it never fails that when people need to redeem accounts for emergency purposes, it is the worst possible time. It is important to note that most of the time and most importantly within their pensions, profit sharing, 401(k) and 403(b), the investment options are usually limited. For investments intended as buy and hold and also within most 401(k) and 403(b)s where client can't make very many changes - try to stay away from the funds that are constantly traded or that have a lot of market timers, hot money funds, etc.

Look for consistent performance and "plain vanilla" stuff – investments that you can really buy and hold.

What to Watch Out For

➢ Try to avoid fads and certain sectors even though they sometimes seem appealing. We pay the managers to pick the right sectors. They are the investment gurus; we are the advisers who are managing them, but not doing their job for them.

➢ The more aggressive you get, the more active/intense the management required. For investments above the moderately conservative level, the best strategy is to either pick a fund with a good consistent long-term performance, preferably with same manager, or pick a manager independent of any of the funds to select the funds and watch and monitor them.

➢ Don't be misled by short term numbers. Especially pay attention to the difference between geometric and arithmetic compounding and how dramatically losses impact long-term performance. I like the bulk of the variable money in the solid investment area such as balanced, growth and income, equity income, blue-chip stock, dividend-paying stock funds.

➢ Inherent in the structure of the investment pyramid, it is important to build from the bottom up and most importantly not be top heavy. The pictorial looks rather like a tree and not a house, but I can best describe it in terms of a mansion-type house. The emergency fund is the foundation, the fixed accounts and conservative municipal bond funds are the base, the balanced funds are the first floor, the growth and income/equity-income/dividend-paying stock funds the second floor, the growth the third floor, the international the fourth floor, the small cap/emerging growth the penthouse. I want to have more on the bottom than on the top so it does not tip over. Controlling the volatility improves the long-term compounded return and most importantly the doctor's investment experience. For the fixed accounts I use money market, CDs and fixed annuities and under very special circumstances fixed life insurance. For the variable portion I use mutual funds or a combination of mutual funds and variable annuities.

Taking the Time

One of the most essential elements to keep in mind when developing a wealth strategy tailored towards clients in the medical profession is the standard timeline. The initial analysis takes about 6 to 8 weeks. And the complete process actually takes about one full year, with the major portion being accomplished during the first 3-6 months.

Ongoing needs, reviews and services are a lifetime process, particularly if the doctor needs practice consulting. This is becoming more and more common due to the constant changes in medical practices. For example, many solo practitioners are now employees or partners in a partnership. Partnerships seem to constantly change. There is a significant movement of doctors from one type of employment to another.

In the end, doctors, just like any other, must have a long-term commitment to have a chance at success.

M. Eileen Dorsey, CFP, EA, MBA, MSFP is a CERTIFIED FINANCIAL PLANNER practitioner in private practice. She is President of Money Consultants Advisory, Inc., a Missouri registered investment advisory firm and Money Consultants Services, Inc. a registered broker-dealer – member NASD. She specializes in retirement planning for professionals.

Ms. Dorsey received her undergraduate degree from the University of Missouri. She earned a Master of Business Administration degree (Beta Gamma Sigma Business Honor Society) from Southern Illinois University. She received the CFP certification from the College for Financial Planning and is a graduate of their Master of Science in Financial Planning program with specialized training in retirement planning. She received the enrolled agent license from the IRS.

Ms. Dorsey is a NASD Registered General Securities Principal and Financial & Operations Principal thru Money Consultants Services, Inc. Money Consultants Services, Inc. exclusively provides broker-dealer and insurance support services as necessary for her clients. She is the Past-Chairperson and Past-President of the Institute of Certified Financial Planners St. Louis Chapter. Ms. Dorsey is an industry arbitrator for the NASD and American Stock Exchange.

Ms. Dorsey is a continuing education instructor for the St. Louis Community College, prior associate professor for University of Missouri St. Louis, a special educator for the AARP and IRS pre-retirement planning programs and frequent lecturer to various groups including major corporations. She has published numerous articles on financial planning and has appeared on TV and radio (both local and national) talk shows relating to her financial planning expertise. These interviews include but are not limited to the St. Louis Post Dispatch, Channel 4 & 5, USA Today, Kiplinger and Morningstar. She is the author of Lifetime Strategies: How to Achieve Your Financial Goals and co-author of Financial Survival Guide For Natural Disaster Victims. She wrote a weekly financial advice column for the St. Louis Sun. She is listed in "Who's Who in Finance & Industry". She has testified before the United

States Congressional subcommittee on small business and the Missouri Senate subcommittee regarding financial planning regulation. She has been recognized as one of the 120 best financial advisors for doctors as reported by Medical Economics.

Rx For Building Wealth

D. Scott Neal, CPA, CFP

President
D. Scott Neal, Inc.

Working against the Clock

Most doctors readily admit that they lack the time to acquire the knowledge of how to develop a wealth strategy. Time has worked against them in two perspectives. One is the number of hours in the day. From residency to retirement, doctors are perhaps the busiest people on earth; many work around the clock with on-call schedules, hospital visits, and administrative workload all added on to regular patient care.

Secondly, doctors are constrained by the time actually spent in their career. By the time they finish medical school, internships, residency, and fellowships, today's practicing physician will be 32 to 34 years old before they are able to begin to produce an income that will enable any degree of wealth accumulation.

There is an old story that if you can begin saving 10% at age 22, you can likely quit saving at 32 and still have accumulated enough money by age 65 to live well. But if you wait until age 32 to begin, your savings will never stop. However, many busy doctors don't get started with any serious savings program until age 45 or even 50. This wreaks havoc with any lasting wealth building strategy.

Another problem that faces a practicing physician is that much of their wealth is tied up in a professional practice that runs on without a succession plan. A succession plan is actually a written plan to get rid of the business someday and receive some value in return. Presumably it would go to another physician or group of them and could be as a result of disability, death, or retirement. Nevertheless, the business of medicine has significant value if approached properly. Two things are necessary in order to overcome this problem. The first is psychological: the doctor's feeling that the practice would not be worth anything without the physician. While this is probably true for many practices, in others, this is certainly not the case. Steps can be taken early in the life cycle of the practice to build it into a business that will stand apart from the practitioner(s) that own it. The second hurdle to overcome this problem is the physical drafting of the plan along with legal agreements, valuation methods, and timetables.

Developing a Purposeful Plan

A financial planning firm can free the doctor from the time constraints of developing a financial plan. One way this is accomplish is by helping him or her develop a purposeful savings and investment policy that encourages the accumulation of wealth. Doctors are blessed with the ability to make a relatively large income. But in reality, only five things can be done with one's income, regardless of the eventual amount.

1. Pay income related taxes: Federal income taxes, state income taxes, local income taxes, social security and Medicare taxes all combine to take a large chunk out of the resources available to devote to the remaining categories of allocation.
2. Debt service: This is the total interest and principal paid on debts of any sort.
3. Save and invest it: A portion generally gets saved.
4. Give it away: Giving away some of income involves the questions of To whom? When? and How much?
5. Spend it on consumption that will probably increase over time due to inflation.

The bottom line of this analysis is always zero. All income gets allocated into one of the five categories. See our chart:

Cash Flow Calculations

Inflow from All Sources

Personal Earned Income-Client		
Personal Earned Income- Spouse		
Investment Income – Interest and Dividends		
Business Income		
Partnership and Real Estate Income (Net)		
Gifts from Others		
Company Match of Retirement Contribution		
Other Receipts		
Total Cash Inflows	**A**	

Outflow

Income Taxes

Federal Taxes		
State Income Taxes		
Social Security Taxes		
Medicare Taxes		
Local Income Taxes		
Total Income Taxes	**B**	

Debt Payments-Principal and Interest		
Home Mortgage		
Home Equity Loan		
Credit Card Debt		
Investment Debt		
Student Loans		
Total Debt Payments	C	

Total Giving	D	

Savings and Investments		
Reinvestment of Dividends and Interest		
Personal Contributions to company retirement plans		
Company Contributions to retirement plans		
Other Savings		
Total Savings and Investments	E	

Total Consumptive Spending	F	
Total Cash Outflows		
Net Cash Flow A minus (B+C+D+E+F)	-0-	

Only after the allocation of income is considered can one develop a strategy for meaningful wealth to grow. In building wealth it is important to minimize taxes, earn a return that is higher than the interest rate on borrowed funds, earn a decent rate of return on savings, give intentionally, and spend with wisdom.

The Real Starting Point

To begin developing a purposeful plan we work through an exercise that helps the physician discover what's important to him or her about money. This exercise was developed by Bill Bachrach in his book, *Values Based Financial Planning*. Few people ever want to create wealth simply for the sake of creating wealth. The real accumulation of wealth has to be purposeful in providing whatever is important to the individual doing the accumulating.

Next we help the client look at his or her goals. To be effective, the goal must have a name, it must have a realistic timetable, and it must be attached to the values identified in the first task.

Next, we take stock of the current financial condition. In addition to the cash flow mentioned in the five things to do with every dollar, a clear statement of assets and debt is essential. This should be documented at current values for assets and current payoffs for liabilities.

Finally, we also assess the defensive side of the equation by carefully reviewing insurance: disability income protection, death benefit, long term care, property and casualty, and liability protection is a must for most physicians. All these things make up the starting point of the wealth plan.

Diversification Decisions

Usually those with significant discretionary cash flow begin the wealth building process without much thought to the income allocation discussed above or even to developing long range goals that are consistent with their values. Instead, most begin with the investment question of where to invest the savings.

The first rule of making investments is diversification. It is critical that before one decides which investment vehicle is most appropriate to decide how much one will allocate to each of seven asset categories:

1. U.S. Fixed Income Instruments such as Cash, CD's, Bonds
2. Fixed Income Instruments of foreign entities either governments or companies.
3. Stocks of Large U.S. Companies (generally those with more than $8 billion of market value)
4. Stocks of Small U.S. Companies (generally those with less than $1 billion of market value)
5. Stocks of Mid-sized U.S. Companies (those that fall in between the two categories of stocks above.)
6. Stocks of Foreign companies
7. Real Estate and/or Commodity-Linked Securities.

It is likely that nearly every investor should invest some of his or her money into each of these categories. Choosing the right mix of these asset classes is probably the most important decision one can make regarding creating a strategy for building wealth.

The Art and Science of the Portfolio

Finding the right mix of these investment vehicles for one's portfolio is often as much or more of an "art" than a "science," but with modern technological tools, it can at least be approached with some valid statistical tools. These tools should result in a better portfolio than would have been created using experience and intuition alone.

Finding the right mix is always a balance between the investor's need for return and the ability to absorb short term declines in the value of the portfolio without altering the plan.

Through interviews and questionnaires we try to get to know the client's tolerance for short term volatility. It is vitally important to choose a mix that can be sustained for longer periods of time. Basic risk management suggests that the more risk one is able to accept in the short run, the more return should be expected. Otherwise, why take the risk?

Through analysis of the goals we provide a forecast of the financial resources that will be needed (at the time that they are needed) in order to fulfill those objectives. This implies an assumption regarding the expected return on the savings and investment and an expected volatility. A key concept is that two portfolios that average the same rate of return, the portfolio with the lesser volatility will have more dollars at the end of any future period. So we attempt to maximize the return provided by the client's investment while at the same time controlling volatility.

If we have miscalculated the client's tolerance for volatility we will know it as soon as the market moves unexpectedly and we may find adjustment is needed. If adjustment to a more conservative or more aggressive portfolio is needed, we generally recommend that those moves be taken in small steps.

Picking the Right Stocks

There is an old adage in the investment business that goes as follows:

"There are 68 ways to pick stocks and they all work. The secret to building wealth is to pick one of the 68 and learn to live with it, in good times and bad."

If one has paid attention to the need to diversify the portfolio into many asset classes, the payoff for picking the right stocks will not, in the long run, produce superior performance in one's portfolio. Instead, time should be spent in finding the money manager (either mutual fund manager or separate account manager) who can make the individual investment decision. We help the client make those decisions through our analytical processes. For example, it would be far too expensive for an individual investor to do enough research to pick the individual stocks of small U.S. Companies or foreign companies. A professional financial planner will assist the investor in picking the right manager and then deciding when to change managers. A planner will use the entire universe of mutual funds and pick the ones that are least expensive for the client rather than the ones that pay the planner the most, as is often the case with *commission-based* and *fee-based* planners.

Managing the Portfolio Monthly

If the portfolio is well-chosen, meaning that the risk tolerance has been assessed correctly and good managers have been chosen; new data with which to update the portfolio usually becomes available monthly. It is then that the time-consuming analysis should occur. Typically, the process of managing a portfolio will require a few hours per month. Watching the day-to-day price movements of a portfolio usually results in ulcers and underperformance of the portfolio. Over time, if the portfolio has been allocated to all the asset classes mentioned above, it will become skewed to have more of the asset class that is outperforming the other asset classes over some time period. *It is more important to re-balance the portfolio to the chosen allocation than to watch the performance of the individual assets that make up the portfolio.*

If additional contributions are being made monthly to the portfolio, managing becomes a two step process:

1) Use the additional funds to buy the asset class that is underweighted relative to the others at the time of the evaluation.

2) Review the managers and determine if the performance of the manager has lived up to expectations in relation to his or her peer group. If not, find a manger that has a higher likelihood of outperforming peers. As Will Rogers is often quoted as saying, "Find an investment that is going up and buy it, if it doesn't go up don't buy it." Monthly analysis of the manager should be conducted in order to ascertain his or her relative performance to peers. We sell an asset when it has dropped to a predetermined level relative to peers rather than a fixed price level.

Changing Directions

Strategies should not be altered due to the mere passage of time. Instead, one should focus on the objectives set and determine if those objectives are still valid and whether the chosen strategy is moving the investor closer to the goal or further away. As important events such as graduations, births, deaths, or retirement get closer in time, a change will likely become necessary. Traditional wisdom has instructed us that one should hold stocks until retirement and then switch to income producing assets such as bonds or CD's. However more recent scholarship suggests that while one should likely become more conservative in strategy and therefore invest less in stocks and more into fixed income; one should not plan to live solely from dividends and interest earned by the portfolio. Instead the portfolio should still be invested to produce an expected *total return*, including dividends, interest and capital gains taken from selling investments that have done well. Out of that total return a sustainable withdrawal rate should be established that meets the need and will grow with inflation.

Bulls and Bears

The economy is continuously shifting, and there are several different approaches to counter a bull or bear market. A buy and hold strategy in low cost mutual funds will work in a bull market. However as volatility rises, more upgrading of the mutual funds will be necessary in order to find those that outperform their peers. Picking those that will likely outperform becomes somewhat easier when the market is whipsawing.

However, aside from the extremes, I believe there are a number of basic rules for making money in any economy. Above all else, stay invested –

through good and bad times. Try to work with the economy, rather than going against the grain. Insist upon getting value for expenses paid, and always be broadly diversified into multiple asset categories. If you pay attention to these fundamentals, the market swings should not cut as deeply.

A Ten Step Guide for Busy Doctors

1. Identify Values. First, decide what's important to you. In *Values-Based Financial Planning,* Bill Bachrach suggests that the question be posed, "What is important about money, *to me?*"[1] Then when that question is answered with X, ask it again with "What is important about X, *to me?*" Keep going until nothing further comes to mind.

2. Identify the financial factors at the starting point. That will be cash flow, assets, debts, insurance, etc. Assets should be listed at their current market value and broken into the following categories: Tax-deferred investments such as retirement plans and Educational Savings accounts, Taxable investments such as brokerage and bank accounts upon which taxes must be paid on current income, and Personal Assets such as residences, cars, jewelry, etc. that are not likely to be sold in order to fund long term goals. Debts should be listed at their current payoff amount. All cash inflows for the current year (year to date actual numbers plus an estimate for the remainder of the year) should be accumulated and the taxability of each inflow should be determined. Earnings should be included at gross levels, not

---

[1] Bacrach, Bill, *Values-Based Financial Planning: The Art of Creating and Inspiring Financial Strategy;* Aim High Publishing, 2000.

take-home. Remember to include any gifts or one time payments to be received.

Taxes should be estimated using this year's rates. Don't forget to include social security up to the maximum level and Medicare Tax on all earned income.

Debt service should be listed to include all payments on debt, but excluding escrow amounts for things like property taxes and insurance.

Savings should be listed including the amount of money that is withheld from gross income for retirement savings in 401k or other retirement plans provided by employer.
Giving should be allocated at some level consistent with your values.

Finally, what doesn't go into one of the four categories already listed can assumed to be spent on consumptive items. It is this number that determines the spending necessary to support a particular lifestyle and it is this number that will go up with inflation. At a 3% level of inflation, this number will double in approximately 24 years. At 4%, the doubling will occur in approximately 18 years. This helps to establish a rough idea of the spending needed to maintain a particular lifestyle in retirement.

3. Identify goals, determining a time frame for accomplishment and quantifying each one. Then find the connection to the values found in the first step.

4. Assess risk tolerance. In other words, ask "How much can my portfolio decrease in value over the short run (say one year) in order to achieve long term results?" We use an online tool produced by Finametrica and found at www.finametrica.com

5. Choose a portfolio mix that will likely meet that risk tolerance. Make sure that it is broadly diversified into multiple asset classes. Our firm has developed benchmark portfolios of exchange traded funds in order to assess the relative performance for different portfolio levels.

6. Determine if the expected return provided by that portfolio will be sufficient to fund the goals identified in step three. This is done with portfolio optimization software that is widely available; however all software is not created equally and small variations of inputs may produce dramatically different results. Use software that is updated with fresh data regularly.

   Our firm subscribes to data supplied by Ibbotson Associates of Chicago, IL as well as that company's optimization software. We chose Ibbotson because of the wide acceptance in the industry. They may be accessed via www.ibbotson.com

7. If the portfolio does not fund the goal, adjust the goal and/or the portfolio. Keep in mind that adjusting the portfolio risk/return characteristics at this stage and living through the declines in the adjusted portfolio are two totally different things. It's much easier to adjust the portfolio while taking a view to the future, but much harder to live with the downturns that inevitably occur when a more aggressive portfolio has been chosen.

8. If an actively invested portfolio is desired, an upgrading strategy will be necessary. Upgrading mutual funds involves a selling strategy that dictates, ahead of time, when the fund will be replaced by one of its peers. Our firm uses an upgrading strategy that rank-orders the selected mutual funds in each asset class. Once the rank has been established we invest new funds into the top mutual fund of that order. When the mutual fund drops below the 25th percentile of the ordered list, we sell that fund and replace it with the fund that is now number one.

8. Determine ahead of time how much to save each month, quarter, or year and make the investment occur as automatically as possible. For example, have it withheld from each paycheck or withdrawn from the bank account each month. Increase the amount from time to time until it's truly noticed. Only then consider cutting back to the former level of saving.

Now, review the cash flow chart developed in step three above. Try decreasing your spending by a set amount next month and have that money deposited into a cash account at your brokerage firm. Next, increase the amount by a like amount in the following month to see if it is missed from your checking account. If it doesn't crimp lifestyle, increase it again and again until it is really felt. Once that level is reached, cut back to the previous level. This will result in your family saving more money and spending less. Now calculate at the expected rate of return, what the additional savings can mean in 1, 3, 5, 10, and 20 years. This would be a good time to review the values arrived at in the first step.

9. Review the whole process at least annually by looking at what you expected to happen versus what actually happened.

Scott Neal is the president of D. Scott Neal, Inc., a fee-only firm that specializes in helping clients make sound financial decisions. He holds MBA and Master of Divinity degrees and has concentrated his service in the areas of estate, retirement and investment planning since 1986. He has been a CPA since 1981, and has been designated a Personal Financial Specialist and a Certified Financial Planner. Scott was recently selected, for the third time, as one of the country's best financial advisors for doctors by Medical Economics. He is a frequent speaker and writer on financial planning topics. Scott is frequently heard as a financial planning commentator on radio and television. You may reach him at scott@dsneal.com or by calling 1-800-344-9098.

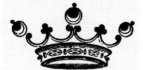

Prescription for Financial Success

William Barton Boyer

President
Parsec Financial

Squaring the Medical Profession with a Sound Financial Plan

Because of their high income and high intelligence, many doctors are handicapped. They think the high income will always be there. Simply put, it won't. Earned income stops for everyone at some point and investment income needs to take over. Being as intelligent as they are, they think a quick analysis is sufficient, or they simply follow a winning trend that their friends are hot on. If this is the only strategy in place, trouble is ahead. Also, scammers know doctors are good targets, as they are often willing to make quick decisions on things they may know little about. In the financial realm, swinging for home runs often hits air and leads to disaster. However, when following a carefully-constructed and goal-oriented wealth strategy, medical professionals can easily pave a wise plan for the future.

Goal-Oriented Stratagems

I'm a big believer in goal setting. In life, what you see is what you get. So, in financial planning, I believe in setting high, realistic goals and then, step by step, taking the actions necessary to attain these goals. Your subconscious is always guiding you to where you will end up. If your conscious goal is simply to "get through the month," then that's about all that will happen. If you are a productive high income person in the medical field, $20,000,000 or more by age seventy is not unrealistic. There are plenty of people in society, including a few doctors, with $50,000,000 or more. And down the road why shouldn't you be one of them? I believe that using the goal-oriented approach to money management is the only way to achieve these successes.

When I am working with a client to help them develop a targeted strategy for accumulating wealth, I encourage them to fully understand where they are financially at present and then adopt a goal-oriented approach to their money management. To steer them into thinking in these goal-oriented terms, I generally have them ponder a few key questions. To set the future goal, the main factors to consider are:

> How much do you have now?

> When do you want to retire?

> What spending level do you want in retirement in today's purchasing power?

> How much can you save annually?

> How is the money going to be invested and what is a realistic return expectation?

If at the starting point, the client has defined a very specific goal, it makes the process of devising the best investment vehicles for achieving this goal far easier.

Do You Want to Be Independently Wealthy?

Securing a means to be independently wealthy would have to be the ultimate goal which a doctor would likely seek for the years after his or her own retirement. Reviewing Appendix form A ("Do You Want to Be Independently Wealthy?"), it takes about 36 years from a zero start with a 15% savings rate of pre-tax income and a 100% equity allocation. Why would you choose 100% equities when most in society counsel 20%-30%-40% fixed income? Well, there has *never* been a 30 year period in U.S. history, not even in the period from 1902-1932, when fixed income has beat equities.

From 1984 through 2002 the return on the S&P 500 was 12.2% compounded annually. DALBAR, Inc. and the Bogle Investment Center found that the average equity mutual fund returned 9.6% annually, while the average equity mutual fund investor earned 2.7% annually during the same period by attempting to outperform the overall market. They do this by going from the cold fund to the hot fund, and when the hot fund turns cold, they go back to money market, etc., (market timing).

So, since market timing is a failed approach, what good is the lower return fixed income allocation going to do for you? It will lessen volatility. However, while downside volatility is diminished, there is generally more upside volatility than downside, so there will be less money in the future as a consequence of less volatility. And less money as you enter retirement means less spending ability against that money. You can spend $500,000 annually (5%) from a $10,000,000 portfolio. If you have only $5,000,000, a spending rate of $500,000 (10%) will jeopardize the principal.

If you spend more than 5% annually from whatever you have, as a beginning spending rate, you approach or exceed the return expectation. The math is very simple; if you spend more than you make you will run out of money. Who's going to call the kids when that happens? Which kid are you going to call? Choose a proper retirement spending strategy that guarantees you won't run out of money. If necessary, lower your expectations so you won't overspend your ability.

predicting terrible equity returns going forward? Equity prices rose about 50% in the next 18 months! 5%, 50% - they got the five part right, just missed the zero.

The Wrong Way

When developing a strategy for profiting in the markets, above all, the cardinal rule is not to commit to market timing. Destroying emotions for investors are always fear and greed, and in a sense, market timing is a combination of both. You're not saving enough, so you need more than market returns, and want to be in the market when it's going up but out when it's going down, fearful of a decline. Three out of four years the market is positive, so it is a three-to-one odds bet against you to be successful in finding that one negative year. To find two negative years correctly without making a mistake is then a fifteen-to-one odds bet against that being done successfully. With those odds, you're better off discarding market timing altogether. What you want is all the upside. And to get that, you have to suffer all the downside. Negative volatility, if you are properly diversified, is simply the price to pay for more money. And as more money is certainly the proper outcome, forget market timing. Preying on the greed emotion, you need more than market returns. You are setting yourself up for trouble ahead.

Another wrong approach is to maintain hedge funds. They are simply high cost mutual funds that can sell short as well as go long, use leverage and charge 4-5% annually with incentive fees added in. You can count on 4-5% underperformance over time compared to the S&P 500. Sure, you could get lucky and pick a great one or you could pick one that goes broke. For example, Long Term Capital Management, the hedge fund with Nobel Prize winning managers, in the end, actually lost it all. Don't

Over the last twenty, thirty and forty year periods ending Decem...
2003, the S&P 500 has enjoyed compounded annual returns of 12...
12.16% and 10.58%, respectively. Never in U.S. history have forty...
returns been far from 10% compounded annually. Projecting s...
market returns at 10% compounded annually is not unrealistic for in...
funds or a low cost investment counsel with a smart approach. High...
cost approaches should deduct excessive fees from the return expectatio...
For example, a fee relationship of 2% annually should project at 8%...
instead of 10%. Also, each 10% allocation to fixed income should reduce...
the return expectation by .50% annually.

For example, a doctor beginning at age thirty with a $120,000 income...
should then set a retirement goal of about $8,000,000. If they don't want...
to work thirty-six years but still want the $8,000,000, they'd have to save...
more than 15% of pre-tax income as the tradeoff.

The Effects of Market Volatility and the Destroying Emotions

This strategy, involving the portfolio mix described, should not change
during wildly up or down markets as we've seen over the last ten years. Of
course, investors will want to stay well diversified between large, medium
and small companies, growth and value, and it's also wise to invest around
10-15% internationally. Above all, the main thrust of this goal-oriented
strategy is to keep adding savings and take the long-term view whenever
possible. And don't let big name personalities persuade you to differ from
this approach either.

In late 1999 the destroying emotion was greed, but in late 2002 it was fear.
Remember deflation, a weak economy, Pakistan and India set to exchange
nuclear warheads, and so on? Remember many investment expert...

trust industry statistics on returns. Mark Hulbert, a well-known mutual fund performance expert, says that most stop reporting as they prepare to close or are going broke, so these dismal numbers don't get in the composite return. His research found 5% annual underperformance versus the S&P 500. I don't want any of that for my clients! Nor should you want any of that for yourself

The Right Way

After delving into all the wrong approaches to developing a strategy for profiting in the markets, I believe the most important step in the *right* direction is to choose the right asset allocation. My personal strategy is to invest in 100% equities, very well diversified. Set the right savings rate, 15% of pre-tax income from a zero start if you have thirty six years, and then be patient and avoid market timing. With this strategy in place, you should also plan to become debt free prior to retirement.

Another recommendation for the long term perspective is to consider investing in real estate as an alternate vehicle. Income producing real estate is competitive to the stock market, and with proper use of leverage, it can deliver even better returns. We certainly favor professional office ownership. Vacation real estate can be excellent as well, plus a lot of family fun. However, don't become real estate poor (too much house) – this is the type of real estate that actually jeopardizes saving what is necessary to accomplish independent wealth.

Retirement Spending Strategies

How should one spend in retirement? To gauge this for your personal circumstances, it's helpful to review two historical examples (Appendix C and D). 1965 (Appendix C) is the "bad look," review as it starts when the Dow Jones was 1000 and didn't pass 1000 again until 1983. You retire just before the worst decade financially since the Great Depression. To track this example, begin spending 5%. Each year that 5% indicates a higher number, spend more. Each year it doesn't, spend the same as the previous year. Never spend more than 10% so that you never jeopardize your money. You could never run out of money as you'd always have 90% left over! While it could be a *lower* number, you could never actually run out. How nice would it be to start spending $50,000 from each $1,000,000 – and you should have many millions – go through the 1973-1974 crash, go through the 1987 crash, go through the 2000-2002 crash and then spend $511,632 the 39th year?

From 1975 (Appendix D), missing one of the once a generation crashes, how nice would it be to start spending $50,000 and increase spending to $873,574 the 29th year? That is 87.3% spending of the original investment. Or, you could be in treasury bills all this time and be spending less than 1% on the original investment. Life is full of choices!

Or, you could use a Monte-Carlo simulation. Start with 60% equities and 40% fixed income. Begin spending at 5% or $50,000 on your $1,000,000. Increase spending 3% annually to offset for annual inflation. Then based on thousands of variables you have an 80% chance of not running out of money. Or, in other words, you'd have a 20% chance *of* running out of money. ANY chance of running out of money is not acceptable. As you enter a distress period like 1973-1974 or 2000-2002, spending 3% more every year jeopardizes your money! This is dollar cost averaging in reverse (see Appendix E). In my opinion, this is simply nuts and should be flatly rejected as illogical.

Shrewd Habits to Build Until Retirement

Habits are hard to break. One healthy habit to develop then is fully funding retirement account opportunities. I believe in only incurring debt on appreciating assets such as real estate. Be in the habit of paying cash for depreciating assets, such as vehicles, boats, furniture, etc. It's also critical to realize that leasing is simply a 100% financed transaction, so don't lease vehicles. Early on, when you don't have much money, buy used vehicles. Or, make a one time exception buying a new car with a three year loan. Keep the car six years, saving up in years 4-6 to pay cash for the next car. Credit cards are fine, but only to the extent that you pay the balance in full each month. Vacations are also great, save up and pay cash.

Finding an Advisor that Fits

Interview several to find one you feel is best qualified and one that meets your needs with a reasonable cost structure. In this case, good quality financial advice really doesn't cost; it pays.

One of my clients once referred their mother to me. She was mad at the world it seemed, and especially mad at me—who knows why, I just met her. She proceeded to tell me her life story. She and her husband were married in the 1930's and made all their own financial decisions; no outside counsel was wanted. They both worked outside the home, which was unusual in those days. They saved a high percentage of their income for 45 years, but they never touched the stock market because they never wanted a negative return. They retired in 1980 with $300,000. The husband died in 1981 and in 1982 the wife bought a five year CD yielding 15%. Life was good – after all, $45,000 of investment income plus social security was fine in 1980. But five years later, the new five year CD rate was 8%, and by the time she came to me five years after that it was 4% (about where rates are now!). She was devastated and unwilling to do anything different – habits are hard to break. She died a year later, bitter and unhappy. This couple's story is a sad one to relate, especially since it has an ending that I believe could have been remedied so very easily. This couple did one thing wrong – they chose the wrong asset allocation. They should have chosen 100% equities and bought Minnesota Mining, Merck, Philip Morris, Coca Cola, Eastman Kodak, etc. Then in 1980 they should have begun spending along the 5-10% strategy I've outlined. For starters, they probably would have lived a lot longer. The Mayo Clinic did a study that concluded positive, happy people live 20% longer. Instead of spending $12,000 in 1995, spending 5% from an all equity portfolio would have been about $750,000. When she died 5-15 years later her daughters would have inherited, even with estate taxes, many millions instead of $150,000 each. There most likely would have been sizable charitable contributions too.

Steps to Success in Any Economy

1) Commit to a high level of success. Put these ambitious goals in writing, long term, intermediate term and short term, and then review them regularly. List the assumptions necessary to accomplish these goals, and then take action. And when you make mistakes, learn from them and take *corrective* actions.

2) Continually expand your education. Plan for job changes, but aim for minimal time between jobs that could disrupt savings.
3) Use debt cautiously; plan to be debt free in retirement.
4) Live within your means, save 15% of your pre-tax income, but don't be a miser.
5) Be positive, not negative. Be charitable, doing random acts of kindness each day, and balancing your life between work, family and friends.

Bart majored in business at Arizona State University and is a Certified Financial Planner. He has been selected by both "Worth" and "Medical Economics" as one of the best financial advisors in the country and was featured on the cover of 2002's July/August 'Best Financial Adviser's' "Worth" issue. He has appeared on ABC's "Good Morning America" and Fox TV's "Fox on Money." He has been quoted in "U.S News and World Report," "Newsweek," "Bloomberg Wealth Manager," "Kiplinger's Personal Finance," "The Wall Street Journal," "USA Today," the "Dallas Morning News" and others. He is the founder (1980) and President of Parsec Financial, a fee-only financial planning and investment counsel firm with offices in Asheville and Charlotte, North Carolina, serving more than 770 clients and managing $560,665,000 as of December 31, 2003.

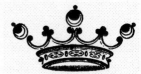

Rehabilitate Your Financial Plan

Mary McGrath

Executive Vice-President
Cozad Asset Management

The Initial Exam

The first thing one must do in establishing a wealth strategy is to become familiar with the client. This entails asking detailed questions about financial goals and objectives, obtaining information about the family, thoughts about retirement, any financial obligations concerning parents, and other issues which should be addressed. It can be described as an informal "getting to know each other" session. This is similar to a patient's initial exam. Prior medical history must be disclosed along with gathering current health information before the initial exam can begin. Once the financial "exam" is completed, a financial statement must be prepared. The financial statement is the starting point. The financial statement lists the financial "vitals" of the client.

Obtaining Test Results

The financial statement lists investments as a whole or in one or two categories such as a joint investment account and a retirement account. Before a financial diagnosis can be made, more specific information must be obtained. All investable assets should be broken down into general asset allocation categories such as cash, fixed income, equities, or real estate. If commodities or other investment vehicles are used, the categories may be expanded. In regard to equities, a more detailed exam is necessary. The equities should be further divided into large cap stocks, medium cap stocks, small cap stocks, and international equities. In a portfolio of individual securities, the equities should be further classified by sectors. One can use the sectors included in the S&P 500 index. This is a way of obtaining further information in order to provide the most accurate diagnosis.

The final diagnosis must take into consideration short-term goals and objectives as well as long-term goals and objectives. Short-term goals may be as simple as an addition on a house, buying a larger house, or a major vacation. Long-term goals are things such as college planning and retirement planning. Determining where one is and where one wants to be lays the groundwork for determining the appropriate prescription that must be written to achieve financial health.

Avoiding Setbacks

Preventive measures should be put in place in order to avoid a major financial illness. In the medical field, vitamins, correct eating habits, and exercise are advised in order to avoid a serious health problem. The same can be said in regard to finances. Potential risks might include the disability or death of the major breadwinner. It could also include a major lawsuit or loss of employment. What happens if you are treating a patient for cancer, and suddenly he or she acquires severe heart problems? The plans to defeat the cancer are then derailed by the problems associated with the heart. Financial objectives can also be derailed if risks are not addressed. If you are a surgeon, what happens if you develop an illness such as Parkinsons, and can no longer operate. Or what if you are involved in a lawsuit, and the judgment stretches beyond your insurance limits, are your personal assets at risk? A prescription must be written to protect from these financial possibilities. Adequate life and disability insurance should be in place. Perhaps long-term care insurance is needed. In addition, asset protection strategies should be used.

Taking Your Temperature (for Risk)

Before writing the final prescription for the financial health of the client, the client's temperature of risk tolerance must be taken. Telling a patient who has a fear of leaving her house that she should go to the mall and walk every day is probably going to fall on deaf ears. In the same way, advising a client who cannot tolerate a decline in her portfolio to invest heavily in stocks is also the wrong prescription. One of the best ways to determine risk tolerance is by completing one of the many questionnaires that have been prepared just for this reason. Questions are answered with a numerical value given to each answer. The answers are then totaled with the numerical result determining the risk tolerance of the client. These types of tests are more accurate than asking a client to verbalize their risk tolerance as most clients don't know their own risk profile.

Financial Prescription

Once all of the tests have been completed, the financial prescription can be written. In a medical case study, you start with the vitals, you interview the client for medical history, you inquire about eating habits, exercise, and stress. Questions are also raised about symptoms – where does it hurt? What is the pain like? Tests are ordered and the results studied. At the end, a diagnosis is made. A financial plan is no different. The financial prescription will include specific steps that need to be taken in order to achieve the financial goals. The steps may include a regular investment plan, a change in current investments, protection of assets, and strategies to avoid pitfalls. The financial prescription should provide the client the best opportunity for good financial health.

You Don't Cut Off a Hand Just Because It Hurts

It is important to invest with long-term goals in mind to avoid short-term changes that can negatively affect overall performance. Once the financial prescription is determined, an investment policy statement (IPS) should be written. An IPS is used to keep emotions out of investing. If a patient comes to you complaining of severe pain in his or her right hand, you don't solve the problem by removing the hand. You solve the problem by trying to determine what can be done to reduce the pain. When a client's investment portfolio decreases due to a downturn in the market, the solution is not to sell the equity portion of the portfolio in order to eliminate the pain of watching the portfolio decline. The answer is to determine what can be done to decrease the decline. An IPS reduces emotional decision making. In the IPS, the financial goals and objectives are spelled out as well as the client's risk tolerance. The IPS also describes what investment vehicles are appropriate as well as defining an overall asset allocation strategy. It should address how investment choices are made, and what criteria are used in changing investment vehicles. A reporting procedure should also be laid out.

Self-diagnosis usually does not work. The patient is too close to the problem. A patient may have recently had a relative who died of cancer. Therefore, every pain he or she experiences is perceived to be cancer. The same is true for investors' portfolios. Every downturn in the market may spell doom to an investor. Every time his or her portfolio decreases, he or she fears a loss of money and bankruptcy. The investor fears he or she will not meet his or her financial goals. The result is a knee jerk reaction and a pulling back from the stock market or making a change in investment vehicles at the wrong time. Studies have been done showing investors are their own worst enemy. One way to avoid this is to return to the IPS before making any changes in the investment portfolio. The IPS should give the client a clear view of his or her investment portfolio, and thus avoid market timing errors as well as performance chasing.

The investment policy statement will identify the appropriate investment vehicles. It might also state what investment vehicles will not be used. For example, one may determine that the appropriate investments are those that are liquid. And yet when confronted with an investment that seems almost too good to be true, a client might decide to invest even though the investment is in a closely held company with no liquidity. By going back to the investment policy statement, the client should be able to refocus on the original financial goals and objectives and make a decision not to change investment strategy.

The investment policy statement should help to protect one from his or herself.

Diversify, Diversify, Diversify

When a patient comes to you and asks what should be done in order to maintain good health, you don't recommend one vitamin – say Vitamin A. It is the same with investments. No matter how much one might believe that a particular sector such as technology is the best sector for the next twelve months, one should not invest 100% in that sector. Medicine is not an exact science. Nor is investing. Diversification allows one to achieve financial goals by providing more predictable returns. Some investment choices will be right, but some will be wrong. Therefore, diversify. No individual stock should represent more than 5% of an equity investment portfolio. Strategies should be developed to reduce any overweighting in the portfolio. Diversification is a way to avoid the risk of a financial failure. Doctors in particular need to be aware of the benefits of diversification. The easier stocks to buy are the ones with which one is most familiar. This means a doctor's portfolio many times gets overweighted in healthcare stocks. This overweighting means an underweighting or elimination of other sectors. Doctors have excellent earning potential. They have the power - they have the income to drive the financial plan. There is no reason to be overweight in a sector and run the risk of financial failure. Diversification allows the doctor to use his or her earning power to build financial wealth.

Just Because You Feel Good, Don't Neglect the Annual Exam

Patients are told to get an annual exam regardless of how they feel. Men should be checked for prostrate cancer even though no symptoms exist. Women should have mammograms. Portfolios should also be monitored even though the overall return is acceptable. One does not need to spend a significant amount of time managing the portfolio. At least annually, a complete financial physical should be done. The allocation of assets should be compared with the investment policy statement. The financial statement should be reviewed to determine if the net worth is increasing. Mutual funds should be reviewed for changes in investment objective or management. Bonds in the portfolio should be monitored to determine if there has been a change in the credit rating of the company. Individual stocks should be monitored to determine whether or not the initial criteria are still being met. A portfolio left on its own is very unlikely to meet the financial goals and objectives for which it was intended just as an individual who never sees a doctor is not guaranteed to stay well.

Financial Rules to Live By

The seven most important factors to consider in making money in any economy are:

1. Stay diversified.
2. Start saving early.
3. Remember over the long term, stocks will outperform bonds.
4. Remember over the short term, stocks are more volatile than bonds.
5. No one can achieve long-term success reacting to short-term trends.
6. Return to the IPS before making changes in the investment portfolio.
7. You will make a bad investment. Forget it and go on.

These tips are no different than the medical tips given to patients as a way to live a long healthy life – tips such as exercising often, eating healthy foods, getting enough sleep, avoiding stress, etc. By following these simple medical rules, a patient is less likely to incur serious health problems. Likewise, an investor who follows these rules is less likely to experience financial problems.

The Diagnosis Should Fit the Patient

If a patient comes to see you and is diagnosed with stage 4 cancer, you don't prescribe exercise and vitamins with the promise of a long and healthy life. Much more drastic measures are needed. If a patient comes in with an inoperable brain tumor, you don't tell them everything will be fine. The same is true with finances. A financial plan should be attainable. If you decide to start saving for retirement at age 60, and you need $1 million by age 65, you will need to save over $13,000 per month. This will not be possible if you earn $200,000 per year. If you are a doctor earning $150,000 per year and have six children between the ages of 8 and 16 and decide to send them to an Ivy League college, saving for college is probably not an attainable goal. The goals must be consistent with the client. The financial prescription must fit the patient. In order for success to be achieved, the financial goals must be realistic.

Mary McGrath, a Cozad executive vice president and certified financial planner, has been providing sound financial advice for more than a decade. Her primary focus is estate and retirement planning for clients of high net worth or high income, including professionals, physicians, retirees, widows, and divorcees. She helps clients define plans designed to help them achieve their financial goals, then implements those plans by furnishing access to sound products in line with their risk tolerance. Through consistent effort and outstanding service, Mary has built a solid base of satisfied clients, and referrals from them continue to expand that base. She is also a registered representative with FSC Securities Corporation. Mary graduated with highest honors from the University of Illinois with a bachelor's degree in accounting. She received a national honor for scoring in the top 1/10 of 1 percent on the exam for certified public accountants, and was a tax partner in a national accounting firm before joining Cozad in 1985. Mary's professional affiliations include membership in the American Institute of CPAs, the Illinois Society of CPAs, the Estate Planning Council, the Executive Club of Champaign County, and the Financial Planning Association. Mary was named in the 1998, 1999, 2001, and 2002 issues of **Worth** *magazine as one of the 250 Best Financial Advisors in the Country. She was also listed in the July 1998, August 2000, and December 2002 issues of* **Medical Economics** *magazine as one of the 150 Best Financial Advisors for Physicians. Both magazines based their designation on the advisor's education, experience, accomplishments, practice size* *and scope, clientele, and compensation method. The nominees were provided by financial professionals and associates around the country.*

Also a dedicated community volunteer, Mary has served as president of the Champaign West Rotary Club, the Estate Planning Council, the Central Illinois Women's CPAs, the Executive Club of Champaign County, and the University of Illinois Quarterback Club. She has been a board member of the Carle Foundation Hospital, Community Foundation of Champaign County, the local YMCA Foundation, the Champaign County Chamber of Commerce, and the United Way of Champaign County. In 1995, Mary was honored with the Athena Award for Professional Businesswoman of the Year at a ceremony sponsored by the Champaign County Chamber of Commerce.

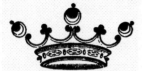

Physician Financial Planning for Wealth Preservation

Wesley D. Bigler &
R. Allen Freeman, Jr.

President; Certified Financial Planner™
Financial Network Corporation

Targeting Physicians' Individual Needs

Over the past several years Financial Network Corporation has worked with physicians to help them protect their assets, manage their wealth and plan for retirement. Physicians, we have found, are a special breed of client. Their advanced education, high incomes, extravagant lifestyles, high self-images and lack of time make their financial planning needs unique. When looking for a Financial Advisor, doctors are typically seeking a firm that has a high degree of integrity, has a proactive approach to solving financial problems for doctors and understands and specialized in the specific needs of physicians. Because of their high-level of education, they expect more from the professionals they choose to work with.

Education and experience are also factors that are important to physicians. Certified Financial Planner (CFP®) Certification is thus an indispensable criterion for a financial planner, as it indicates that he or she is educated, experienced and has high ethical standards. CFP® professionals are highly trained individuals who must complete a comprehensive course of study at a college or university that offers a financial planning curriculum. CFP® professionals must also pass a comprehensive certification examination based on the financial planning process, tax planning, employee benefits and retirement planning, estate planning, investment management and insurance.

The CFP® Board's Code of Ethics and Professional Responsibility set forth the standards of ethical responsibilities to the public, clients and employers. All CFP® practitioners must abide by the Code of Ethics and agree to provide planning, advice, and services that are objective and put the client's interests first.

In many ways, we follow the same method of inquiry and resolution as medical professionals. When doctors ask for a medical history, we gather facts about a client's financial history. Following the same analogy, as doctors observe and record patient symptoms, we record client concerns and goals. In both cases medical tests or financial calculations are performed, ultimately resulting in a diagnosis; doctors diagnose a physical illness and financial planners determine a client's financial need. Both professionals offer a solution – whether in treatment or a comprehensive financial plan. And both "patients" are likely to need to return to follow-up on the plan that was originally prescribed. With these similar modes of analysis, it should be a lot easier to understand what it takes to construct a financial plan favoring doctors.

Asset Protection

Because many doctors live excessive lifestyles, it is important they are able to maintain that lifestyle no matter what may happen in life. Many doctors either own their own practices or are partners in a larger practice in effect making them business owners. It is not only important to protect assets for the doctor, but for the doctor's family. Any protection they have must be adequate to cover the loss of business were they made unable to practice medicine for a period of time or indefinitely. Assets can be protected using a number of methods.

Understanding and planning for claims of liability in the case of an accident is one of the key needs of doctors that financial planners deal with. All practicing doctors understand the need to protect themselves from malpractice lawsuits. Many, however, do not realize that they may be at a higher risk for personal lawsuits because of the perception that they are wealthy. For instance, a prominent ophthalmologist has a summer dinner party. As the guests mingle beside the pool one of the guests turns her ankle when stepping from the patio on to the grass. That injury would normally be covered by any standard homeowner's policy. The injured guest knows that the homeowner is a doctor and assumes that he has enormous wealth and decides to sue, claiming loss of work, additional injuries and pain and suffering. The general perception is that doctors have "deep pockets" and can afford to pay anything. There are even individuals whose main goal is to take from those who have, and doctors often fall prey to these types of individuals. Therefore it is crucial for doctors to enact several different measures in order to protect themselves, and they have several options:

> *Liability Insurance and Umbrella Policies*

It is important that physicians maintain umbrella policies that cover all of the insurance options maintained by the physician. Umbrella insurance is designed to give added liability protections beyond the limits of a single homeowners, auto or business liability insurance. The insurance is designed to be used when a liability claim is more than what a single policy can cover.

Business assets also need to be protected. Doctors who own their own practices or are partners within a larger practice are essentially business owners and must consider the protections needed for their businesses. They must also ensure that a business liability does not affect their personal assets.

> *Limited Liability Partnerships*
For medical practices, Limited Liability Partnerships (LLP) allow the physician and their business partners to operate the practice without exposing themselves to personal liability in the event that the business is held liable for something that occurs in the office

or within the confines of the business. Additionally, one partner in the business is not liable for any malpractice that does not involve that partner.

➢ *Limited Liability Corporations*
A medical practice may form a LLC (Limited Liability Corporation) to take ownership of the practices expensive medical equipment. The equipment is then leased back to the practice. If the practice is sued, the equipment is protected from the lawsuit because it belongs to a separate legal entity. The practice may establish other LLCs for additional assets owned by the practice.

Insurance

Most physicians need either more Disability and Life insurance coverage or specialized policies that help them to ensure that their specific needs are met – like a disability policy that pays a physician who can no longer practice as a physician, even if he is able to work in another profession. Physicians also need to protect their practices and partnerships from death or disability.

➢ <u>Disability Insurance</u>
Because of the physician's high income, it is extremely important to have protections in place that will guard against loss of income due to injury or disease. Disability insurance offers protection from temporary or permanent loss of work due to health issues.

It is important for any financial firm handling the planning for doctors to understand that standard disability insurance may not be appropriate for those in the medical profession. Own-occupation disability insurance provides salary protection in case of an injury or illness that prevents the doctor from practicing medicine – even if he or she is not prevented from participating in another profession. For instance, a surgeon may lose the use of her right hand and no longer be able to perform surgery, however she can still teach at a medical school. Own-occupation disability insurance will pay her doctor's salary even though she may be earning near the same salary as a professor.

The Doctor's financial advisor must also understand that any physician working in a medical practice must also have disability coverage that will protect the business. In order to be fully protected, the practice must maintain disability insurance that will take care of any loss of income to the business during the recovery period or in case the partner is unable to continue working as a physician.

➢ *Life Insurance*

Any professional understands the significance of obtaining life insurance to ensure that his or her family is taken care of in case of death. In order to maintain the family's current lifestyle, it is important that a physician have adequate life insurance coverage. A financial advisor familiar with the specific needs of doctors can help the professional to understand the amount needed to supply the family with ongoing income. As an example, $1,000,000 in life insurance may only yield $50,000 in annual income to the family.

Again, it is important to protect the medical practice as well as the business. Partners can establish a Buy/Sell agreement within the partnership. For traditional partnerships, in the event of a partner's death, the ownership of the business is transferred to the heirs of that partner. A Buy/sell agreement establishes a life insurance policy naming the business partner as the beneficiary with enough coverage to cover the cost of the deceased partner's portion of the business. The living partner can then purchase the remaining portion of the business from the other partner's family.

Tax Planning and Estate Planning

Proper tax planning can help a physician to maintain his or her lifestyle while ensuring that business and personal taxes do not pull more from the physician's salary than is absolutely necessary. Utilizing Family Limited Partnerships or asset-balancing in the financial planning process are both great strategies to implement, which a skilled financial advisor can walk the physician through.

> *Family Limited Partnership*
   A family limited partnership (FLP) is a business created by an agreement between a physician and certain members of the family. It is typically used when an owner of real estate or a business wants to centralize and consolidate management and to reduce estate transfer costs by shifting future increases in value to younger generations. The FLP is a business and financial planning device that can combine business operational planning, personal tax planning, transfer of family wealth, and business succession planning, all under one flexible arrangement.

   Although this is a highly effective method for simplifying tax planning and reducing estate transfer costs, there is a degree of risk involved; Family Limited Partnerships must be carefully established and maintained, for if it appears that the discounts are too large, tax penalties may be assessed. It is important that these agreements be maintained by a firm who specializes in these types of strategies for physicians in order to ensure that all agreements are made within the boundaries of tax law.

> *Asset-balancing*
Asset-balancing is the act of taking personal property such as a personal residence or second home or jointly held bank accounts and ensuring that it is titled as tenants in common rather than joint tenants with rights of survivorship (JTWRS). For instance, most people own their homes or even second homes as JTWRS. Assume a married couple owns a home worth $1,000,000 and it's titled as JTWRS, such a title arrangement could create a substantial estate tax burden on the surviving spouse. Alternatively, if the house were held as tenants in common, $500,000 of the property is titled in her name and $500,000 is titled in his, then only half the total value would be included in the surviving spouse's estate and the other in the deceased estate, thus enabling to couple to take advantage of the unified credit.

Wealth Management

Essentially, wealth management is centered on planning for the future by ensuring that current income will help to fund future events such as retirement, college tuition for children, care for an aging parent, care for a special-needs child and long-term medical care. Any highly-paid profession needs a certain level of financial planning for retirement. Other professionals, however, do have more flexibility in how they handle their retirement. An accountant or attorney can become semi-retired for ten years and continue an accounting practice on a part-time basis. Corporate professionals can continue with consulting businesses and in many instances actually use retirement to become entrepreneurs.

Physicians, on the other hand, find it far more difficult to practice medicine on a part-time basis. The cost of malpractice insurance alone can be prohibitive to allowing the physician to practice part-time. Most established practices and hospitals are not going to be willing to pay the malpractice insurance for a physician that is unable to bring in enough business to offset the cost of the insurance.

Of course, a physician who retires *can* go on to another profession. However, even this option is difficult. Even though physicians are highly-educated and intelligent individuals, their education is so specialized that it is often very difficult to use that in another profession. Furthermore, many times a physician's high self-image as a doctor will simply not allow him or her to move into another profession.

Therefore, early and structured wealth management is especially important for those in the medical profession. The answer is establishing an effective Wealth Management Strategy that will ensure that the amount of yearly income after retirement is at or above that income maintained before retirement.

Preparation Questions for Physicians

When a physician is broaching the idea of developing a new, comprehensive wealth strategy, it is vital for to be very thoughtful about answering a number of financial questions that the advisor will inevitably ask. Preparing oneself for these questions in advance not only saves time, it helps the financial advisor and the client become better acquainted during the initial consultation. A few questions to consider are:

Financial Goals

> ➤ When do you expect to begin withdrawing money from your investments? For how many years will you be making the withdrawals?

> ➤ You must consider several types of risks when investing. All of these risks mean you can lose money in your investment. You cannot reduce one type of risk without assuming another type of risk. What portfolio mix are you comfortable with:
>   - A high chance of short-term declines in value but with an opportunity for portfolio growth significantly greater than inflation rate.
>   - A moderate chance of short-term declines in value in a portfolio that seeks growth that is moderately greater than inflation rate
>   - A low chance of short-term declines in value but with the chance for portfolio growth slightly greater than inflation rate.
>   - A very low chance of short-term declines in value with a portfolio that only grows fast enough to keep pace with inflation.

> ➤ Are you willing to lose larger sums of money in the short term if you can enjoy potentially higher returns in the long term?

> ➤ Are you more focused on increasing returns, reducing risks or a combination of both?

> ➤ Assume that you invest $100,000 in a portfolio that is expected to have high long-term returns and high short-term risks. The portfolio's value grows to $120,000 in the first year. If your

portfolio lost all of its previous gains and some principal in the next month (dropped to $85,000) how would you react?

- Not concerned, maintain the investment
- Somewhat concerned, shift to slightly more conservative portfolio
- Very concerned, shift to much more conservative portfolio.

➢ After a three-year period, if we were to meet and review your portfolio, what results would lead you to feel satisfied about your progress?

➢ Are there any asset classes or investment vehicles you do not want in your portfolio?

➢ Describe the best and worst investment you ever experienced.

Personal Goals

In addition to addressing financial matters, a good financial advisor will also seek to uncover some more personal information concerning your lifestyle and personality. Knowing what is most important to you outside the realm of money can be a great indicator to how you might react to certain scenarios or to what decisions might best coincide with the remainder of your life and interests. Spend considerable time thinking about how you might answer some of these questions that pertain to your lifestyle:

➢ What are you accumulating wealth for?

> If you had all the money you needed, what would you do with your life?

> What past achievements are you the most proud?

> If you were going to die tomorrow, what would you most regret not doing?

> What financial things do you currently have that you appreciate the most?

> What are some things that you set out to obtain that have not done so?

> If you were to look back over your life today, what, financially, will you have been most grateful for accomplishing?

> What are you most proud of financially?
> Do you expect to be responsible for your parents' care in the future?

Building upon the Consultation

The initial consultation is a face to face meeting that determines the personal and business financial goals of the client. This consultation, which would generally last anywhere from one to two hours, is the first step in the pathway to developing a successful wealth strategy and lays the foundations for the rest of the relationship between the physician and the advisor. These two parties review the client's current financial status and address any questions and concerns that may arise. The outcome of the meeting is that the advisor will present suggestions for the client's consideration and discuss the development of formal written financial plan is developed.

When the physician client begins the process with Financial Network Corporation, the first step is to complete the Client Profile. The Client Profile includes questions that help the advisor to more accurately determine the physician's current financial situation, future plans and financial and personal goals. Significantly, the profile not only focuses on the financial, but the personal, asking questions such as: "What past achievements are you most proud of?" and "What are some things that you set out to obtain and have not done so?" These questions help the advisor get a more complete picture of the physician's desired future.

The consultation appointment is the first chance for the physician and the advisor to get to know one another. The advisor will use the opportunity to share the wide range of services offered by Financial Network Corporation with the physician. During the initial consultation, the advisor also goes through the process with the physician and helps him or her to understand every step that needs to be taken in order to achieve the financial goals that have been set. Mutual understanding is thus one of the key elements that make for a successful consultation. If the physician decides to pursue a wealth strategy with this particular advisor, he or she then leaves the meeting with the task of gathering both personal and business information for the upcoming data appointment. The physician should be busy for the next one to two weeks with collecting and organizing the following types of information:

➢ Financial statements

➢ Wills and Trusts

> ➢ Insurance policies

> ➢ Partnership agreements

> ➢ Other investment information

Data Appointment

The data appointment is a two to four hour meeting scheduled after the initial consultation, when a physician has had a chance to gather all financial information including all current investments, wills, insurance policies, corporation papers, etc. At this point, the advisor assesses all current information and begins the development of the formal plan.

The purpose of the data appointment is to review all of the physician's current financial information. The advisor will also discuss other personal information with the client and ask questions that will help him to get a better understanding of all of the client's needs. It is at this point in the development of the wealth strategy when the specific needs of the doctor become important, and must be recognized and thoroughly discussed. It is imperative that the advisor understand all factors that may affect the doctor's financial well-being and what it will take to maintain the physician's lifestyle through the changes that naturally occur during the course of life and after retirement.

Because of the high incomes of doctors and the active lifestyles that many of them maintain, it is important that the advisor ask all of the appropriate questions during this phase to ensure that the physician is aware of their own financial needs. Some of these questions include:

➢ Does the client have children?

➢ If so, what are the client's education goals for his/her children?

➢ Does the client have a special-needs child?

➢ Does the client have elderly parents or could there be any future issues with parents?

➢ Does the client's spouse have any special needs?

It is also important to understand that for most individuals, lifestyle habits do not change unless some drastic change occurs in their life. Those who live frugally will continue to do so after retirement. Those who spend a lot will continue to want to do so after retirement. The advisor should thus model their plans on the current status of spending and saving ratios for the physician and his family.

The physician will also bring the reviewed Investment Policy Statement and completed questionnaire to the Data Appointment. The purpose of the Investment Policy Statement is to establish reasonable expectations and guidelines for the investment of the physician's portfolio and set forth an investment structure detailing permitted asset classes and the expected allocation among asset classes. The Investment Policy Statement also creates the framework for a well-diversified asset mix that can be expected to generate acceptable returns at a suitable level of risk. In addition, this statement continues to encourage effective communications between the advisor and the client. The statement provides the client with an explanation of the following factors that affect the portfolio:

➢ *Time Horizon* – the length of time before the physician will be drawing money from the portfolio

➢ *Risk Tolerance* – the ability of the physician to tolerate fluctuations in the market

➢ *Asset Allocation* – ensuring that the portfolio has the proper diversification to ensure optimal growth

➢ *Rebalancing Procedures* – the process of periodically reviewing the portfolio and making changes when life events occur, needs change, or changes in the market occur

➢ *Investments* – types of investments that can be used to create the optimum solution for the physician

➢ *Duties and Responsibilities* – responsibilities of the advisor and the physician in order to ensure that all of the physician's financial needs are met

➢ *Portfolio Determination* – summary of the time horizon and risk tolerance based on the answers to the questions in the questionnaire.

The questionnaire that accompanies the Investment Policy Statement asks a series of questions that help the advisor to better understand the physician's Time Horizon and Risk Tolerance.

Timely Plan Development

After gathering and reviewing all of the physician's information, the advisor uses computer models and his or her own vast experience to develop a financial plan for the physician. Based on the answers provided in the Investment Policy Questionnaire, the advisor uses a scoring model to determine the physician's Time Horizon Score and Risk Tolerance Score. The plan includes all financial information and recommendations including:

- ➤ **Cash Flow Analysis**

- ➤ **Asset Protection Analysis**

- ➤ **Tax Planning**

- ➤ **College Funding**

- ➤ **Insurance Analysis**

- ➤ **Investment Analysis**

- ➤ **Retirement Planning**

- ➤ **Estate Planning**

The intention of the Plan is to ensure that the doctor is able to maintain the same level of lifestyle even when the unexpected occurs. It takes into account scenarios for what may happen if the doctor is unable to continue practicing medicine, one or both of the parents are deceased, planning for college costs for the children and the event that funds may be needed in order to take care of an elderly parent or parents, just to name a few of the scenarios. Once all of these factors are considered and the plan is developed, carefully tailored to the physicians' individual needs, it is presented to the client.

An ideal timeline for developing this type of comprehensive wealth strategy from the initial consultation to the implementation of the plan could last anywhere from 2 to 8 months. Of course, all of the decisions made during the course of the plan development are with the physician. The physician chooses when to call Financial Network Corporation, determines how long it will take to gather all of the data needed, makes the decision about moving forward with the plan and the decision about implementation. Now, taking into consideration the busy lifestyle of the physician (both personally and professionally), and the tendency for many in that profession to procrastinate when it comes to personal and financial matters, the ideal timeline for developing the wealth strategy could grow considerably. Once all the information is in however, the plan rests with the financial advisor.

Plan Presentation and Implementation

Once the initial workup of the plan is completed, the advisor presents the plan to the client. All of the information is wrapped up in a summary that includes all of the findings and recommendations for creating a fully supported financial plan.

The physician and the advisor meet again to review the plan summary and make investment determinations based on the information provided in the plan summary. The role of the Financial Network advisor is to use his experience working with the physicians and his or her knowledge of their unique financial needs to make recommendations based on the information provided by the physician. Finally, it is then up to the physician to determine which of the recommendations that will best suit her financial needs.

The financial plan summary also includes all investment options that gives the physician optimal return on her investment and meets the physician's time horizon and risk tolerance needs. Investment options may include any of the following:

> Large Cap U.S. Equities

> Small/Mid Cap U.S. Equities

> International Equities

> Emerging Markets Equities

> Domestic Equity/Bond Blend (Hybrid)

> International Equity/Bond Blend (Hybrid)

> Real Estate Investment Trusts

> U.S. Government Bonds

> U.S. Corporate Bonds

> U.S. High Yield Bonds

> International Bonds

> Municipal Bonds

The plan summary also outlines recommended insurance policies, recommendations on wills and trusts, recommendations on steps to take to help protect business assets and additional resources to help the physician achieve a balanced financial plan.

After the client has reviewed the plan summary and made decisions, a process which can span from one to four weeks of careful consideration, the plan is implemented. Additional professional services are recommended (i.e. legal, accounting, insurance, etc.). And once the physician determines which of the recommended steps that will be taken, this portion of the plan is also implemented. This may involve establishing trusts, moving investments to more or less conservative stocks or bonds and taking steps to ensure that appropriate asset protection is in place.

After all of the planning and preparation, it is important that the plan is carried out. The purpose of the financial plan is to ensure that all affected parties are taken care of no matter what may happen. There are many causes of an unsuccessful plan and all of those have very definite consequences.

The plan may fail because the client:

> Procrastinates – A doctor has a vacation home worth $850,000 on the coast. His family vacations there and rents it out a good part of the year. His goal is to retain the house in his family for future generations to enjoy. There are two issues with the way he has the property ownership established.

1. He owns it joint tenancy with right of survivorship (JTWROS) which will create a substantial estate tax burden on his wife and family.

2. Owning the house JTWROS and using it as rental property opens him up to tremendous liability in the event he is sued by a tenant, potentially costing him his life savings.

The Doctor is advised to change the type of ownership in the property and put it in the name of a separate entity, but he puts that off and subsequently continues to leave himself open to legal liability.

➢ Implements only part of plan.

➢ Doesn't follow investment policy statement – A doctor invests in too risky investments, i. e. too much tech stock, or too much in money market and not participating in the market. Many investors got out of the market in 2002 and had money on the "side lines" in 2003. This caused them to miss a significant rise in all of the investment markets.

➢ Constantly changes their mind – I once had a doctor who had an estate tax issue and we set up a life insurance policy owned by a trust to create the liquidity to pay the hundreds of thousands of dollars in death taxes and provide more money to the surviving wife and children. After a period of time the doctor cancelled the policy to save the premium dollars, ultimately costing his family substantially in lost wealth transfer that will now go to the IRS.

➢ Is looking for greener pastures, or "the next best deal."

Staying Current with Periodic Reviews

Once all elements of the plan are in place and have been fully implemented, the physician and advisor meet once again to review all aspects of the plan and address any issues, concerns or questions that the client may have since he or she has seen the practical effects of the plan. At this point the physician and advisor also determine when such reviews should take place (whether annually, semi-annually, or quarterly) and what upcoming life events will trigger reviews (such as a child moving out of the house or a parent moving in).

In order for the financial plan to remain current and effective, these periodic reviews are required. The advisor and physician should budget one to two hours for the review, during which the advisor and physician mainly assess the following:

> ➢ Are the current investments continuing to meet the physician's needs?

> ➢ Are all assets being appropriately protected?

> ➢ Are current insurance policies enough to cover the physician's needs should something happen?

> ➢ Have any changes occurred that could affect the physician's future financial plans?

Once the review is complete, changes may be required to the plan in order to continue to maintain the effectiveness of the portfolio. The physician and advisor will also discuss any future events that may require additional reviews.

Financial Resources Geared to Physicians

The Financial Network website www.FNCOnline.com provides a wide array of information that can help individuals assess their own financial situations including past newsletters, articles, information of other resources (attorneys, accountants, banking services, career counselors, etc.) and information for business owners.

The Prosperous Retirement Guide to the New Reality by Michael K. Stein, CFP (EMSTCO Press, Boulder, CO, 1998) is an excellent resource for physicians embarking on the road to a profitable wealth strategy that will pay off for their retirement. Michael K. Stein provides an abundance of information for anyone who desired to have the retirement of their dreams. It also includes practical information on planning for that retirement and managing the plan according to the parameters previously outlined in this chapter.

Wesley D. Bigler, a Certified Financial Planner, has been involved in the financial service industry since 1983. As the President of Financial Network Corporation, a full service financial planning company, Wes strives to meet the needs of individuals, business owners, pre-retirees and retirees. He focuses on money in transition, 401(k) plans, estate and retirement planning.

Extensive background and knowledge in the financial and retirement planning fields allow Wes to provide outstanding service to his physician clients. While focusing on long-term relationships, Wes commits himself to in-depth planning and investment advice. Through consistent effort and a reputation for integrity and professionalism, he has built a solid client base and expanded his business through referrals from satisfied clients and other professionals.

Sharing his expertise, Wes conducts seminars for major Atlanta businesses, colleges, numerous associations, community schools and churches. He has also been quoted in major publications such as **Smart Monday, Worth, Financial Planning, New Choices, Atlanta Journal Constitution, USA Today** *and* **National Business.** *Wes is a frequent guest on the CNBC "Money Club," and the New York Based Fox News Channel's "Fox on Money." In the fall of 1997, 1998, 1999, 2001, 2002 and again in 2003, Wes as named one of "The Nation's Top 250 Financial Advisors" in the September issue of* **Worth Magazine.** *Wes was also featured as one of "The 120 Best Financial Advisers for Doctors" by Medical Economics Magazine in 2000 and 2002.*

Wes graduated cum laude with a degree in political science/history from Utah State University and also received his master's degree in business from the American Graduate School of International Management. Wes is past President of the Financial Planning Association, Georgia Chapter.

Active in his community, Wes has been and elder at Mouth Paran Church of God, a committee member for Boy Scout troop 200, and Chairman of the Board of Directors, Cobb Pregnancy Services. Wes resides in Smyrna, Georgia, with his wife Jan and his children, Tyler and Lauren. In his leisure, Wes enjoys camping, tennis, skiing and golf.

FNC has successfully served hundreds of individuals and businesses through its structured and thorough financial planning process. The achievement of security and wealth is reached through the customized design and implementation of individualized creative concepts and strategies. Founded in 1978, Financial Network Corporation, a registered investment advisor, operates under the rules and regulations of the Securities & Exchange Commission.

FNC manages the work of creating and maintaining financial plans for clients through its extensive network of both in-house and outside professionals. FNC believes financial success cannot be achieved unless the plan is expertly implemented. Investments are handled through Financial Network Investment Corporation (FNIC), a national securities broker/dealer. Insurance and other risk management needs are met through a full-service general agency, representing many of America's top-rated companies. FNC's affiliations with several attorneys, accountants, banks and other similar professionals round out the extensive client services available.

R. Allen Freeman, Jr. CFP® is a Certified Financial Planner™, and has been involved in the financial services industry since 1999. Allen also strives to meet the needs of individuals, business owners, pre-retirees and retirees. Extensive background and knowledge in the financial and retirement planning fields allow Allen to provide outstanding service to his clients. While focusing on long-term relationships, Allen commits himself to in-depth planning and investment advice. Through consistent effort and a reputation for integrity and professionalism, he is growing his client base and expanding his business through referrals from satisfied clients and other professionals. Prior to joining Financial Network Corporation (FNC), Allen was affiliated with another financial planning firm in Atlanta.

Allen focuses on money in transition, 401(k) plans, estate and retirement planning. Sharing his knowledge, Allen is an instructor at Kennesaw State University teaching the estate planning course for those enrolled in the Certified Financial Planner ™ CFP® program. He has conducted many workshops and seminars with leading companies in Atlanta and been featured on an 11Alive News segment (WXIA-TV, Atlanta) focusing on financial planning. In order to meet the wide range of his clients needs, Allen is registered in securities, is licensed in life, health, accident and sickness insurance and is a registered investment advisor representative with FNC. Allen obtained a B.B.A. in finance from Georgia State University in 1989. Prior to the financial services industry Allen was involved in commercial and investment real estate in Atlanta.

He is currently a member in good standing with the Financial Planning Association and is a member of Hillside United Methodist Church in Woodstock. Allen lives in Town Lake in Woodstock with his wife Carrie and three girls, Keela, Macey and Abigail. The Freeman's enjoy vacations to the mountains and beach and Allen enjoys sailing, cycling, tennis and golf.

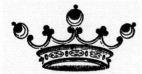

It's More than Money

Paul K. Fain, III

President
Asset Planning Corporation

Targeting Family Physicians

According to B. Joseph Pine Jr. and James H. Gilmore in their book, The Experience Economy, Americans want to have an experience with the products and services that they consume. Even in the process of building wealth, investors want to experience peace of mind, the thrill of growth, and the comfort of financial security. With this trend in mind, my financial planning firm looks and operates a lot like a family doctor's office. In fact, we intentionally make an effort to create the experience of an old country doctor. So, not coincidently, our client database is mostly family physicians. Everything about the way we practice is familiar to them – examination, fact-finding, diagnosis, treatment plans, bedside manner, personal attention, etc.

In addition to emulating the experience of the friendly physician's office, we also base our approach to wealth management on the family doctor's holistic model. We view wealth as an integration of financial, family, social, career, and physical well-being. Certainly, as it has been said, "Money makes the world go 'round," but who has not also heard, "Money can't buy happiness."

Physicians are some of the hardest working professionals on the planet Earth. They train for years and years; they bear tremendous responsibility for the health and well-being of numerous families; and they are passionate about their calling. Nonetheless, the face of healthcare has changed enormously in the past decade, and, many physicians are weary and frustrated. For example, in my client review meetings, family physicians, whom once described themselves working until they died, now ask me when they will be able to retire. Unfortunately, the contemporary demands of the healthcare industry have significantly lowered the job satisfaction of many medical practitioners. With regard to personal wealth strategies, family physicians want to know two things:

> Figuring out how to transition to financial independence (retirement) within the chaotic health care environment, to retire early or at least reduce their workload or to leave their "career" job to pursue working on their own terms. Specifically, doctors now want to know how much money they will need in their nest eggs and how to successfully accumulate those funds.

> Auditing their portfolios and investment strategies. The volatile markets of the past 10 years, including one of history's worst bear markets, have left many open wounds. As much as anything, I feel that many investors need or want to be "resold" on the merits of investing in the stock market as a means to build wealth.

A "Big Picture" Overview

The answers to specific financial questions should always be first viewed in the context of the individual's, or family's, integral financial plan – keeping the proverbial "horse" (the financial plan) in front of the "cart" (the wealth). It may be surprising to know that most families don't have a written plan for the accumulation and management of personal wealth.

The development of an initial financial plan, or wealth management strategy as many call it today, typically requires about one quarter, or three months, from start to finish, which would then be followed by periodic updates and reviews. To begin, I recommend a series of hour-long "family meetings" to discuss each family member's lifelong dreams, current goals and specific objectives. It is not unusual for some tension to occur between contrasting or even opposing objectives. Hopefully, through honest communications and healthy compromise, a family can prioritize financial objectives and the functional utilization of their resources.

Over the course of several days, or weeks, the family should pull together relevant financial data needed for analysis and review: tax returns, savings and investment statements, insurance policies, estate planning documents, etc. Not only is this information necessary for planning, it is incredibly beneficial to engage in streamlining and organizing the data and creating a central repository for future reference. The actual number crunching, projections and scenario building may require several weeks to a month or more. Depending on the individual or family's skill sets, some homework and skill building may be called for, if not also the assistance of a financial professional (see reference list at end of chapter). There now exists a plethora of "how to" books on wealth management as well as numerous financial planning and portfolio management software programs available in retail outlets and on the Internet.

The implementation of a wealth strategy is normally the longest part of the process. Over the course of six to eight weeks, accounts are opened, assets are purchased, liquidated, or consolidated, and regular deposit schedules are established (preferably by automatic payroll or bank draft). Wealth protection issues are addressed as insurances are applied for and contracts are issued. Wealth management and distribution actions are discussed and implemented with the support of an estate attorney in a series of meetings.

Finally, in review and maintenance mode, I recommend that a client invest several hours per week into advancing his financial literacy via financial magazines, books, and the Internet. Each month and quarter, several additional hours should be invested in updating portfolio information and reviewing asset quality and portfolio allocation data.

Annually, a more comprehensive review of the individual's or family's overall wealth strategy might require the better part of a day, or a series of two to three hour investments.

The process of building wealth is as much art as it is science. The "art" is more behavioral than anything else. Our family history, personal experiences, relationships, and current financial situation contribute to form our own unique money personality. Which personality and behavioral traits lead to successful wealth accumulation?

After surveying 1,115 millionaires around the country, authors Thomas J. Stanley and William D. Danko co-authors of The Millionaire Next Door, came up with seven common denominators among those who successfully build wealth:

> They live well below their means.

> They allocate their time, energy and money efficiently, in ways conducive to building wealth.

> They believe that financial independence is more important than displaying high social status.

> Their parents did not provide economic outpatient care.

> Their adult children are economically self-sufficient.

> They are proficient in targeting market opportunities.

> They chose the right occupations.

Successful accumulation of wealth, in all of its forms, is about living consciously and with a purpose. This means being in control of your money and your life. When you save your money rather than continuing to spend it, you buy yourself control. And, then you have a say in how you'd like to spend your time.

With money saved and invested, you can live for years without earning money, or you can at least afford yourself the luxury of working part-time. These millionaires have created lifestyles and jobs that are meaningful to them because they took a look at the big picture and made choices accordingly.

Realistic Expectations

To help my family physician clients develop their strategies to accumulate financial wealth, we first take them through a process of drilling down from their big picture life goals to specific objectives, then to concrete time frames and dollar terms. At that point, we can shift their focus back out to portfolio-influencing decisions such as "how much do I need to save each year?" or "what long-term rate of return does my portfolio need to achieve to accomplish my goals?" When we are working together to find the answers to these questions we find that the wealth management process is also about managing expectations. Too often, our expectations of wealth, of portfolio returns, of a specific asset, are based on what we see and hear in the media.

In my experiences with clients, some of the best laid long-term financial plans and wealth-building strategies are often derailed, or even hijacked, by short-term influences – such as these hyped up media reports. Sensational headlines or passionate opinions shared at the office water cooler or the backyard grill can skew an investor's expectations and prove fatal to a well-constructed financial plan. When these dramatic influences push emotional triggers, such fear or greed, and coincide with monthly investment account statements showing dramatic gains or losses, the stage is set for an investor to ignore their long-term goals in response to the news flash of the moment. For this reason, I repeatedly emphasize how the client's big picture life goals should determine the plan's expectations of the portfolio and how "success" should be defined by the attainment of specific objectives, not a co-worker's inflated braggadocio.

Constructing the Portfolio Mix

In other words, the financial planning process should be the foundation of the portfolio design process. Based on their current financial situation, financial objectives, investment timeframe(s), financial literacy and investment experience, an investor can structure (or restructure) an appropriate asset allocation mix utilizing five or more asset categories.

Our primary investment vehicle for constructing portfolios is the open-end, no-load mutual fund. For most investors, I believe that mutual funds are the wealth-building tool of choice. This amazing wealth-building tool, gives us indirect access not only to money markets, bonds, and equities, but also gives us indirect access to real estate, natural resources, precious metals, etc. In the 1970's and 1980's, our firm offered direct access to these tangible markets, but the results were spotty at best, and often very discouraging. With mutual funds, we hire experienced managers, with research teams to support them. In mutual funds, we are obtaining diversified portfolios of individual securities, at very reasonable costs, with an enormous amount of liquidity and flexibility within our portfolio.

Furthermore, there is voluminous, high quality research available for the selection and ongoing management of mutual funds.

We also utilize individual bonds, fixed and variable annuities, and cash equivalents such as certificates of deposit as clients' needs dictate. Periodically, specific concerns or financial planning issues arise that require a guaranteed or steady income stream, principal protection, or tax benefits, all examples of reasons that we might use an alternate investment vehicle versus a mutual fund.

In our investment advisory service, we manage individual stocks only in more speculative situations such as a concentrated company stock position; or an investor wanting to trade securities more frequently; or a client who simply needs more "stimulation" from part of their portfolio. For example, we might create a separate brokerage account, labeled the "Vegas" account, in which the client trades individual stocks in pure speculation. We partner with them on the research, selection and ultimate disposition of the individual stock positions using reputable stock evaluation tools.

Evaluating a Strategy's Yield Success

I feel that there are subjective and objective, qualitative and quantitative, ways to measure the "success" of a wealth accumulation strategy. On the "soft" or qualitative side of a portfolio, an investor should consider whether or not they feel comfortable with their portfolio's risk level. Do they feel a sense of peace and optimism that their wealth strategy is moving them toward the fulfillment of their life goals? On the "hard" or quantitative side, the advisor must evaluate whether or not the strategy is fulfilling the needs of the client's financial plan. In other words, is it achieving the targeted rate of return? Monthly income? Cash liquidity? Tax benefits?

Investors tend to consciously focus solely on the bottom line - the measurable statistics of yield, appreciation, or tax deductions. But I suggest that this interest is driven by qualitative motives, often unconscious, such as the need to achieve a certain level of status, to retire from a demanding job, or to provide comfort to a family. Learning to recognize and monitor one's "true" metrics of success is a critical component of a wealth strategy.

Focusing on the Long Term

Well-defined goals, and clear measures of success, are powerful allies in the wrestling match with our own emotions. Effectively managing a wealth-building plan often feels counter-intuitive – especially when an investor's goals are long-term, like planning for retirement. Consider the following: investors typically want to buy stocks when prices are appreciating rapidly, not sell them as conventional wisdom holds. Conversely, investors tend to sell stocks when prices are depreciating rapidly, not buy them as the old adage, "buy low, sell high" purports.

Human behavior and prudent investment strategy don't always mix well. A young investor may assume that a bull market will result in the accelerated accumulation of wealth and subsequently an early retirement. Meanwhile, an older investor may react to a bear market by liquidating all equity positions in his portfolio. In reality, both investors have "long term" investment horizons. The young investor, with perhaps 10, 15, or 20 years until retirement, should be focused on long-term average portfolio returns.   The older investor who is currently retired or approaching retirement may still have a 20 to 30 year time horizon to mortality. I often remind my clients, using charts and statistics, that over most rolling five-year periods, and almost all rolling 10-year periods since 1925, stocks have outperformed bonds and bonds have outperformed banks (cash assets)!

The reality is this: short-term planning produces unpredictable short-term results. While, long-term planning, though requiring much more discipline, produces more predictable, steady outcomes that can help an investor reach a rewarding retirement goal.

Learning from a Professional

One of my late father's favorite axioms was "the K.I.S.S. principle – Keep It Simple Stupid" (P. Kemp Fain, Jr., CFP®, who was truly a pioneer in the financial planning profession). In my personal financial plan, I am trying to abide by this maxim; my plan for accumulating financial wealth is simply to invest regularly and take calculated risks. I pay myself first each month (i.e. save) via automatic payroll deduction to my company's retirement plan. I invest regularly in the market through the monthly purchase of a diversified portfolio of stock mutual funds. And, it is as important to me to keep the profits that my portfolio generates as it is to earn the profits to begin with. Subsequently, I include stable asset categories in my personal portfolio mix, including, bonds, bond funds, fixed annuities, and cash/cash equivalent assets.

Also, during wildly up or down markets many investors complicate matters by altering their financial plan dramatically. My personal strategy doesn't change during volatile markets, but my activity levels do! I methodically increase my stock purchases during downturns and I'm very attentive to rebalancing from over-weighted to under-weighted assets during market surges.

Another of my personal mentors, Richard Wagner, CFP, said these timeless gems of financial wisdom: 1) Spend less. 2) Save More. and 3) Don't do anything stupid. To expand on this advice, I try to remember the following:

➢ Spend less than you earn.

➢ Save and invest more than 10% of your earnings.

➢ Include at least five asset categories in your portfolio mix.

➢ Rebalance your asset allocation at least quarterly.

➢ Review investment quality each month.

➢ Follow a disciplined investment strategy of buying points and selling points.

➢ Crisis = Opportunity.

➢ Greed is NOT good.

I frequently share these value statements with my clients and, more importantly, I encourage every investor to develop their own financial value statements – guiding principles for their personal wealth strategy.

The Changing Face of Investing

Every few decades, we find ourselves in strong crosscurrents of economic turmoil, political debate, and global saber rattling. At times like these, a clearly defined wealth strategy is an anchor in our lives – adding stability and keeping us from drifting.

Today, without question, we have entered into a new era for global investment markets, the global economy and the global citizenry. No, I don't believe that the business cycle has been repealed; nor do I believe that bull markets and bear markets are a thing of the past. Quite the contrary, but I do believe that the dramatic events of the past decade have brought us to another tipping point in history, one in which the days ahead are unpredictable. This era may be remembered for a skyrocketing budget deficit, a staggering national debt, troubling health care issues, terrorism against Americans at home and abroad, wars, record low interest rates on savings and debt, soaring personal bankruptcies, and immoral and unethical behavior extending from corporate board rooms to the trading floors of Wall Street. In a few words, the world is marked by uncertainty and hardly more so than in the United States of America. Investment returns are going to be below historic averages for the next five years. Thus, investors with wile and determination are going to be in search of higher yields and capital appreciation opportunities. And sometimes, recklessly so. I think we'll see a new wave of investor speculation, including a spate of alternative investments promising exciting results for hum-drum portfolios.

And indeed, investors and advisers may add new wrinkles to our investment portfolios (or wealth building strategies), but 10 years from now, I firmly believe that the core of our long-term wealth accumulation strategies will still be the same: stocks, bonds, and cash instruments.

Setting Priorities for Physicians First

The absolute first step in establishing an efficient wealth strategy must be to identify and prioritize major life goals. A financial plan without meaning and purpose behind it is like an automobile without a steering wheel. A client's goals give meaning to the accumulation of wealth – financial or otherwise. In my financial planning practice, I go to lengths to help individuals and families define what "wealth" really means to them. The term itself conjures up images of mansions, yachts, and Wall Street. But in reality, we enjoy many different kinds of riches during our lifetimes – work, family, relationships, spirituality, community, and creativity. The wealth of loving family relationships, the wealth of spiritual growth, the wealth of community service, and so on must be factored into the equation to get a full picture.

When we step back from our harried work-a-days of contemporary life, many people are surprised to discover that identifying what they really want out of life is illusive. This can be an extremely difficult exercise for hard-working, highly specialized professionals like physicians. So often, the intensity of their careers when mixed with the resultant high earnings form patterns of personal stress and consumption, living in the moment, and not thinking about the future or about long-term wealth accumulation.

Another pioneer in the financial planning profession, George Kinder, communicates three incredibly effective questions for initial goal-setting in his book "The Seven Stages of Money Maturity." Kinder helps the investor think about what financial decisions they would make if you had all the money you needed, if you had 5-10 years to live, or if you had only 24 hours left to live. In view of these frameworks, a physician should ask him or herself what am I missing in this life?

If you view saving as simply the opposite of spending, how could you commit to it? It's punitive rather than rewarding. To save, you need a goal. Setting goals is both the heart of financial planning and its most difficult task. It requires that you really stretch your mind and think about how you could create a life that's fulfilling. Look inside yourself and reach for your dreams. That is tough stuff. It is much easier to focus on short-term crises and to solve immediate problems, than it is to define your dreams. In addition to George Kinder's thought-provoking questions, I additionally provide the following list of questions to help my physician clients think more directly about their goals when they are seeking to implement a financial plan:

> Do you presently have a wealth management plan?

> Are you on track to achieve your lifetime financial objectives?

> Are you effectively managing your cash flow to build wealth?

> Are you satisfied with your current personal and financial situation?

> Does your current investment allocation strategy reflect your personal risk comfort level?

> Are you self-directed or more of a delegator?

> Do you have strong emotional responses to certain asset categories?

> Are there specific investments in your portfolio that you feel negatively about?

➢ Are there any specific constraints placed on your investment portfolio?

➢ What kind of family life do you want?

➢ How much and what kind of time do you want to spend with your family?

➢ What is most important to you in your living space – size, outdoor space, urban, rural, nearby theaters, sports, a garden, a pool?

➢ What do you want to learn about? What do you need to learn about?

➢ What is it that you most like to do? What do you do best?

Based on a physician's vision of the future and core values, and recognizing the constraints of finite resources, he or she can begin to prioritize primary and secondary goals. In this context, the accumulation of financial wealth takes on deeper meaning. And the question of "how much is enough?" is often much less than imagined before.

Setting a Specific Timeline

So how much *is* enough? A "goal" is a somewhat nebulous thing; it becomes a more concrete objective when it is expressed in terms of years or months, and dollar amounts or regular income streams. With specific metrics serving as yardsticks, a client can begin to track his progress toward an objective, and, ultimately recognize goal attainment. Even unconsciously, humans are motivated by goals. Like the proverbial carrot dangled in front of a horse to move it forward, specific and measurable objectives can be very effective motivators. The opposite is true as well. Lack of vision, goals, or specific objectives can be foreshadowing of financial disarray, budget and debt mismanagement, job burnout and even depression. One of the keys to using objectives to motivate progress is to make them attainable (not unrealistic), to review them regularly, and to be prepared to make adjustments as needed (as opposed to rigid adherence).

Reaching the Number-Crunching Stage

Next, it is vital to take inventory of the individual or family current financial situation and consider obstacles and potential pitfalls. A review of current cash flow – a summary snapshot of monthly or annual income and expenses. And, a personal net worth statement, a summary of current assets and liabilities at fair market value or outstanding balance. Accumulating financial wealth is a process of intentionally shifting money from the cash flow statement to the net worth statement. It begins with creating discretionary cash flow that can be invested for long-term growth. What challenges, predictable or possible, does the client face? Consideration is given to job stability, short-term major expenses, and health concerns. How will taxes and inflation affect the client's financial plan? Wealth management is less a destination than it is a journey. The landscape is constantly changing.

The next step lies in using careful analysis to evaluate planning projections and scenarios. This is the critical research and numbers crunching stage of the wealth planning process: is the client on track to achieve his life goals? If not, what alternate paths might be acceptable? Often in this step, a client must differentiate between wants, needs, and must haves – reprioritizing goals. Physicians are notorious for denying the importance of this step. Their faulty reasoning is that they have enormous earnings potential that will always overcome any shortcomings or mistakes in their wealth building strategies, i.e., a failed speculative investment, or "temporary" overspending.

Physicians also underestimate how much they do need to save to retire comfortably. Ordinarily, most families can retire comfortably with 60% to 80% of their pre-retirement income. Without much thought to a specific target retirement income, most physicians save the maximum tax-deductible amount that their employer sponsored retirement plan allows. As of this writing, that amount is the lesser of $41,000 or 25% of earnings. Unfortunately, in most cases that I see, even contributing $41,000 per year to a retirement plan is not going to be sufficient to replace two-thirds of the income of a physician at retirement.

Comprehending and Delegating an Action Plan

Develop an action plan and review process: who, what, when, how much. In the implementation and review stages of a wealth strategy, an investor must seek education, be motivated, and know when to delegate. Physicians are quintessential take-charge, type-A, quick decision makers. Obviously, this has several major advantages in their personal financial plans. What may be less apparent however is that this behavioral style also has several disadvantages. These intelligent, knowledgeable professionals often have minimal financial literacy – after all, when do they have time to add this complex knowledge to their skill sets? However, many physicians would be the last to make such an admission. This is an important crossroads in the wealth management process for physicians, reaching a point of vulnerability and openness to the knowledge and awareness that they don't have all the answers to their own financial status. Therefore, when it comes to implementing their financial action plan, the key is delegation.

For many investors, and certainly physicians, one of the first "aha" moments of financial self-awareness is the acknowledgment of the individual's worldview of investing. Investors can be segregated by those who believe in the tenets of marketing times, or not; and by those who believe that individual securities selection can produce superior investment performance, or not. Most financial advisers believe that markets cannot be consistently timed, i.e., successfully picking entry and exit points at the most opportune moment; and, they do not believe that individual securities selection will consistently outperform a market benchmark, such as, the Standard & Poor's 500 Index. In contrast, most individual investors believe that they can time markets successfully *and* they have the unique skills required to consistently select outstanding stocks. One of the critical waypoints on the journey of a true wealth management strategy is realizing that building sustainable wealth is a slow and steady process based on long-term investment principles such as asset allocation and diversification via tools like index mutual funds.

Executing the Plan: One Piece at a Time

Armed with the knowledge of how much they need to save each year, what portfolio rate of return will move them toward their lifetime financial goals, and with an understanding about their personal investment philosophy, a physician can begin to implement a wealth strategy. I recommend that an investor tackle no more than two to three action items per quarter – probably choosing the most urgent items or those relating to his highest priority objectives. In my experiences, trying to tackle too many action items at once is a major energy drain and momentum killer.

In contrast, staying focused on a limited quarterly "to do" list provides more immediate feedback, recognizable progress, and serves to motivate the individual and/or family to achieve further progress!

At a point, many physicians appreciate the need to delegate a) the responsibility of acquiring and maintaining financial knowledge, b) the expertise for analysis and planning, and c) the strategies and products of implementation, to an expert. When it comes time for a check-up, physicians have a tendency to treat their own wealth strategies like a patient visit. Due to the time demands on their day, they quickly review a medical chart, scan the patient and engage in some small talk, expertly reach a diagnosis and move to the next examination room. In their personal financial plan, it is prudent to map out a review and ongoing wealth maintenance plan that includes monthly, quarterly, and annual activities including portfolio performance reviews, asset allocation rebalancing, and investment quality decisions. Furthermore, other important wealth strategies include estate and tax planning updates and risk management reviews, i.e., analysis and revision of insurance types, amounts, costs, beneficiaries, etc.

Often, partnering with a financial professional is a very effective path to wealth maintenance, lifelong learning and to elevating personal financial literacy.

Additional Resources

The following websites and books have proved beneficial to many of our firm's physician clients and we continually recommend them.

www.fpanet.org (Certified Financial Planner™ referral source)

www.kinderinstitute.com (life planning resource)
www.morningstar.com (mutual fund research)
www.vanguard.com (online financial planning tools)
www.ssa.gov (Social Security and Medicare information and benefit calculators)

The Seven Stages of Money Maturity by George Kinder
Your Money or Your Life by Joe Dominquez and Vicki Robin
The New Retirementality by Mitch Anthony

Paul K. Fain, III, is a Certified Financial Planner ™ practitioner. He is the president, and a second-generation business owner of one of the country's first independent financial planning firms, Asset Planning Corporation.

Since 1992, East Tennesseans have watched Paul as a weekly financial commentator on the weekend morning news of Knoxville's NBC affiliate. He also contributes a monthly column to the Knoxville News-Sentinel. For the past 16 years, Paul has taught a popular wealth management workshop for the University of Tennessee Personal and Professional Development program. He is a frequent provider of presentations and workshops for organizations such as the Financial Planning Association, the Knoxville Utilities Board, American Association of Swine Veterinarians, United Parcel Service, University of Tennessee, and various State agencies.

Paul and his firm, Asset Planning Corporation (APC), have been recognized as one of the top financial planning firms in the country by publications such as Bloomberg Wealth Manager and Medical Economics magazines. Paul describes APC as a practice that is focused on providing fee-based comprehensive financial planning to individuals and families of East Tennessee. Paul has served as a volunteer on various councils and taskforces for the Financial Planning Association, the largest professional association in the financial planning industry.

Prior to entering the financial planning profession, Paul was with ProServ, Inc., an international athlete management and sports marketing corporation. He also worked in several public relations and marketing positions at two major universities; and, hosted radio and television programs, including, "This Week in Big Orange Country" for the University of Tennessee Athletic Department.

He holds a bachelor's degree from the University of Tennessee and a Masters degree from Ohio University. Paul is a Children's Ministry Director at Two Rivers Church and especially enjoys the teaching and drama aspects of that calling. Paul's family includes wife Tina and three wonderful children.

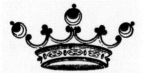

LifeWealth: Achieving True Personal Wealth

Jerry Foster

CEO & Founder
Foster Group

The Impact of Wealth Strategies on Doctors

Foster Group is the only approved financial business partner with the Iowa Medical Society. Physicians comprise approximately 60 percent to 70 percent of our clients. We are a financial planning and investment advisory firm, dedicated to providing unbiased advice to our clients. In nearly every situation, how successful you are at investing has a profound influence on your lifetime cash flow. Investment clients usually have long-term financial goals, including saving for retirement, creating education funds, or establishing a charitable trust.

We work with each client to create an Investment Policy Statement (IPS) that describes *why* he or she is investing and defines *how* funds will be invested to achieve identified goals. This document provides guidance for both the client and the investment advisor. Academic research, as well as our own experience, has shown that clients who take the time to develop an IPS are far more likely to maintain prudent investment discipline in times of high market returns (when euphoria and greed cause people to ignore risk) and during times of bleak economic circumstances (when fear drives people to make damaging short-term decisions).

Major Issues That Investors Must Take Into Account

Investors have to take into account two primary emotions exhibited by clients: fear and greed. Both of these cause people to make decisions based on feelings rather than facts, which is never a good strategy.
Ego also comes into play. Too often people are overconfident and believe they possess the intelligence that will allow them to outperform the markets – something that very rarely happens.

People also tend to react to ever-present media pressure. The major investment media are exceptionally good at convincing investors that they constantly need to be "doing something." Resisting this pressure requires a great deal of emotional strength on the part of investors who may be made to feel as if they are contradicting the advice of "experts."

Developing a Strategy For Accumulating Wealth

Assessing a client's risk profile is an essential tool when developing individual investment strategies. This type of profile describes how someone "feels" about risk as well as how vulnerable plans are to investment risk. Clients should receive a thorough education about the historical performance of different investment strategies, types of investments, and general assets. This education serves as a foundational for evaluating current and future investments.

To help clients develop a strategy that fits their financial goals, you need to help them understand how crucial controlling their monthly cash flow is. Potential investment results are of little importance if an investor can't put funds aside for investment and make certain that they remain invested long-term. You also want to advise clients on how to eliminate and avoid debt. Reducing the interest paid on debt service is the equivalent of a guaranteed rate of return, often at rates significantly higher than those you expect from a long-term investment portfolio. Eliminating debt also potentially reduces additional expenses such as the need for higher levels of life and disability income insurance.

It's important to educate clients about how capturing the return that markets produce over long periods of time, and doing so in a cost-effective manner, is the preferred approach to investing. Helping clients understand that much of what they hear and read about investing is driven by marketing rather than academic research is critical as well.

Once established, an investor's strategy shouldn't change frequently, if at all. Unless the client's financial situation undergoes a change due to significant health issues, marriage, divorce, etc., there is no reason to alter the investment strategy. In the absence of any major life changes, restructuring the strategy suggests that you believe the basic workings of markets have changed or will change; history tells us that's unlikely.

It's good practice to periodically review the performance and volatility of an investment portfolio and how it is matching up with the investor's expectations and comfort level. If a significant variance exists, an adjustment in allocation may be needed; however, this doesn't equate to a change in strategy. It simply means the initial allocation of the account may have been off-target. The same investment strategy can be applied to a portfolio that's more or less aggressive.

Managing a portfolio can actually take less time than investors imagine if an investor accepts the concept that active portfolio management is not only unnecessary but oftentimes counterproductive. An investor should be able to easily manage a portfolio using no more than a few hours a month. Most investors imagine that managing a portfolio involves what they've seen portrayed by the investment media: hours of research to find just the right investment, additional time spent monitoring the investment so it can be bought at just the right price, and even more time making sure that the investment is performing as expected. And if all doesn't go according to plan, investors start repeating the entire process to find the next "right" investment. Academic research, which is not driven by a brokerage firm's marketing department, consistently shows that this model doesn't work effectively for most investors. Consistently capturing the return of markets over long periods will put an investor well ahead of 90 percent of the investors out there.

Strategy Goals

The goal of any strategy should be to provide you with a measuring stick for considering new investment possibilities. Many investors lack an overall strategy. They tend to look at individual investment decisions in isolation and, consequently, often end up with a portfolio that's not diversified enough and that doesn't make much sense when the investor looks at the whole picture. Too often investors try to assess whether an investment appears good or bad in and of itself. They should, instead, be looking at whether adding an investment to an existing portfolio will result in positive change. New investments should be assessed in terms of how they increase or decrease diversification, expected volatility, and rate of return.

Long-term goals might not necessarily affect the strategy that an investor uses but they may have an affect on the allocation of the portfolio. The more lofty the long-term goals, the higher the investment portfolio's required rate of return, all things being equal. And the higher the required rate of return, the more the portfolio needs to be exposed to equities rather than fixed income investments. This scenario might also bring more volatility along the way and a wider range of possible outcomes (terminal wealth). If the goals are high and there's significant ability to invest, it's generally safer to invest more dollars in a less volatile portfolio than to invest less dollars in a more volatile portfolio. The probability of hitting the goal is higher in the first scenario because the range of outcomes is narrower with a less volatile portfolio.

Factors That Affect Investments

Retirement is one of the factors that can affect allocation to a certain degree but it does not necessarily change the investment strategy. Investors sometimes make the classic mistake of viewing retirement as the time horizon of the portfolio. But because of increasing life expectancy it's not unusual for an investor to spend 20, 25, or 30 years in retirement. For that reason, life expectancy should be considered as the time horizon of the portfolio; this almost always argues for a more aggressive portfolio allocation than an investor might believe is needed. Making a portfolio too conservative just because someone has reached "retirement age" exposes them to huge risks many years down the road. Unfortunately, those risks don't become apparent until it's too late to rectify them.

Market changes also do not necessarily affect investments, although that's difficult for many investors to believe. Markets are driven in the short-term almost exclusively by emotion: we feel compelled to act because everyone else is acting, or at least it seems so. Resisting the urge to react - to do something - requires tremendous courage but it's the right thing to do because emotional decisions are seldom right decisions. Decisions based in fact and logic are more likely to produce better results in the long-term. History has demonstrated repeatedly that markets appreciate over time; investors who stay the course during turbulent times profit most often from this premise. Investors can picture the market this way: Say you are riding an up escalator while playing with a yo-yo. The ups and downs of the yo-yo are the equivalent of the wild, daily ride of the markets but the consistent upward path of the escalator is where the market is headed long-term. We have to learn to ignore the yo-yo and focus on the escalator.

Future Changes

In the years ahead the amount of information available to the general public and the speed with which this information becomes available will take a quantum leap forward. Although this should improve investors' results, those pursuing active investment strategies will generally continue to perform below expectations in the markets.

Because of the corporate scandals that came to light during the past few years, more attention will be focused on corporate governance issues. Full disclosure will be required more than ever from individuals and companies providing investments products and services to the general public. The manner in which an individual or firm is compensated for the financial services they provide will become more transparent to the investing public.

Working With New Clients

There are several steps you can take when you begin working with a new client who is considering investment strategies. It's important to assess the client's current circumstances, goals, objectives, and dreams. After ascertaining that information, you want to establish a baseline for where the client is financially and for where they want to go and then create a strategy that focuses on those goals.

To put an investment strategy into action you need to establish timelines and put into place mechanism that will enable you to realize when and where progress has been realized. Measuring progress allows clients to monitor their successes and reaffirm their vision for the future.

For their part, new clients also need to ask themselves some very important questions that can help determine if their investment strategy is in line with their goals:

> Do these recommendations detract from my current quality of life and standard of living, and what are the risks to me and my family if I don't take action today?

> Am I in control of most of the variables and unknowns in the projections, i.e. savings rate, spending assumptions versus tax rates, rate of return?

> How flexible are these recommendations if things don't go as planned? As my advisor, will you be available to help me stay on track, monitor progress, and adjust my strategy to changing conditions and circumstances?

Advice Worth Noting

Successful investing requires planning, analysis, and, yes, perseverance. There are several guidelines you want to follow in order to make the most of your investments.

> *Diversification is the investor's best friend.* Hold a globally diversified portfolio made up of widely diverse asset classes.

> *Participate in asset classes without regard to market timing.* Market timing has never proven successful over long periods of time.

➢ *Don't attempt to beat the market by security selection* ; instead, use asset class investment vehicles to efficiently capture market returns: "be the market."

➢ *Costs matter!* Control costs by reducing internal expenses and minimizing trading, and remember that any reduction in cost is the equivalent of increased return.

➢ *Rebalance the portfolio.* Monitor your portfolio and make changes as necessary to maintain your intended allocation.

➢ *Reduce the costs of building and maintaining the portfolio.* You'll find that this is even more important during years when investments and the economy aren't doing very well.

All of these guidelines will help you choose and maintain the investments that are best suited to you and your lifestyle. It's also essential that you eliminate fear, greed, and ego from your investment decisions. If you let these behavior patterns interfere with your decisions, undoubtedly you will make wrong choices that will, at some point in time, have consequences. Investments can be very rewarding, but they are also very challenging. The people who are most successful in the investing arena are those who think long-term and who are not looking for a quick fix. If you have patience and commitment, you can expect to see returns on your investments and, ultimately, the fulfillment of your present and future goals.

True Personal Wealth

As we have worked with highly successful people, we have found that achieving wealth is a goal that is illusive unless one has clearly defined what wealth looks like.   Defining wealth in the traditional sense includes things like homes, cars, retirement plans and investment accounts. However, it takes on a different look when a person is asked to finish this statement; *Wealthy is the person who...* After reflection, most people will finish that statement with responses like; has meaningful relationships, is healthy, is content, is at peace with their creator etc... This kind of thought process produces a whole different level of personal insight into what really will bring personal fulfillment and satisfaction.

We call this *life*Wealth which is defined as the accumulation of financial, relational, physical, spiritual, and intellectual capital.   Understanding each of these dimensions of wealth and seeing how they are all integrated helps a person see the big picture of life and begin making choices that will put them on the right path of living the life they want.

As planners, we need to help our clients see this bigger picture of planning.   To strategically plan for our financial needs without consideration of the other dimensions of wealth, is incomplete planning. Ultimately most people will measure their success in life by looking at the outcome in each of those dimensions.

So ultimately, we should be helping them answer this question; "How do you want your life to end?"   With your final breath do you want to utter, "What a satisfying, fulfilling, and meaningful life I have lived"?   I don't know a single person who isn't looking for that kind of a life.   What could be more meaningful as a planner than to help facilitate this process for our clients?

Jerry Foster is the founder and CEO of our company, which was founded in 1989. Jerry is a Certified Financial Planner and has written articles for national publications regarding investment and planning matters. He frequently speaks to physician groups regarding life-planning issues and is currently leading the implementation of LifeWealth Planning Services which is an integrated life coaching and financial planning process. He is also a frequent speaker for the CrossTrainers weekly men's group in Des Moines, as well as FamilyLife Marriage Conferences. Jerry is the author of lifeFocus: **Achieving a Life of Purpose and Influence.**

The Foster Group team has been represented on **Worth Magazine's** *top financial planners in American as well as* **Bloomberg***'s top financial planning firms and* **Medical Economics** *top 150 financial planners. More information about The Foster Group can be found at* www.lifewealthstrategies.com.

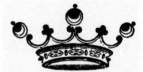

Fixing a Financial Plan
for Professionals

Michael L. Brown, JD, CPA

Partner
Brown & Brown Financial

Financial Plans for Professionals

I would like to focus on two types of individuals who struggle with their personal financial management. My financial planning practice focuses on both doctors and executives; I like to link them because of their many similarities. Both groups are extremely busy and make significant incomes. And as a general rule, both groups have very little experience, knowledge or interest in their finances and investments; they simply have too many other obligations at hand. While it is true that *some* of these individuals are willing to take on these financial planning responsibilities, many times they lack the experience and knowledge necessary for the task, and often make the worst investors. However, with the correct planner and financial preparation in place, these professionals can continue to execute their wealth strategy.

An Influx of Options

I believe the greatest issue and frustration for investors is the overwhelming number of investment options available to them. Add to this their lack of time and experience to analyze and compare their options and this leaves doctors and executives even more discouraged.

There are literally thousands of different stocks, mutual funds, bonds, annuities and other investment products from which to choose. And since the ultimate impact of the clients' investment decision bears directly on their future financial well-being, they are overwhelmed with the enormity of their responsibility to do the best job they can. They know their decisions could very well impact their retirement or the educational funding for their children or simply allowing them to achieve financial use questionnaires to make certain that they have on paper enough information from their client to establish long term goals and objections. Ideally, once the client's goals have been established they *should* be put on paper and then signed by both the investment advisor and the client. Please understand that many of these goals need to be adjusted for risk and reality. A great example of this was with one of my long-time clients who was so bullish with his outlook of the stock market, he wanted to invest 90% of his portfolio in equities. By committing this to writing, he had to really think about his decision. He also agreed to share his Investment Plan with his wife, who was not involved in their finances. Although somewhat ignorant in investment theories, she agreed to review the one paragraph Investment Plan. She knew little about investing, but knew this strategy was too risky for her. It resulted in a heated debate and an eventual compromise with a reduction of their equities to only 65% equities.

The stock took a nose dive soon thereafter. Both were very happy with the decision they had made and they pondered what to do next. Their stocks now represented 50% of their total portfolio and felt a little unsettled and more risk adverse. So we took out their Investment Policy Statement and re-read it. They realized they had agreed to be 65% in the market so instead of selling stocks, they bought more so that the equities represented 65% of their portfolio. Within a year the market rebounded. Stocks now represented 75% of their total portfolio. They called me and we talked. We decided to sell off some stocks that had run up and reduce their stock position to only 65%. They knew they would prevail if they stuck to the plan.

Once a client's goals and objectives have been established, you can then move forward to determine the appropriate asset allocation to best achieve their goal. Asset allocation is simply used in determining the percentage security. They realize the significance of all investment decisions and they want to do the best thing.

Furthermore, they are human – so many individuals suffer from the "greed factor" where they not only want to invest appropriately, but they really want the best investment returns possible.

Most investors think that investing requires you to select the very best stock, then buy it at the lowest price and eventually sell it at the highest price. As a result, the fundamentals, risk and diversification are sometimes glossed over by the novice investor. Thus, the best way to help clients develop long term wealth strategies is through education. Sadly, many investors come to the relationship with good or bad investment experiences, all of which can be difficult to overcome. I am sometimes thankful for the investor who has lost significant money because of his failure to recognize the pitfalls of risk or the failing to recognize the benefits of diversification. At least these investors realize that there is a lot more to investing than simply picking tomorrow's Microsoft.

To educate clients in these areas requires personal face-to-face meetings over an extended period of time. They also must feel a significant level of trust, faith and competence in their investment advisor. Many investors realize that picking the appropriate investment advisor is the key to achieving their financial goals.

Establishing Objectives from the Outset

Once the client has a basic understanding of all the investment landscape opportunities available to them, it is then important to establish the goals and objectives of the client. Again, this process takes time. Many firms of investment assets that will be allocated to the various investment classes such as, equities, income, real estate, and possibly alternative investments. Alternative investments can include hedge funds, collectibles and other more esoteric investments.

Who Can Help

One of the great problems of investing today is that many people in need of investment advice and counsel do not necessarily select the best and the brightest. Investment managers with favorable long-term performance, and respected academic credentials and years of experience in the industry can not be accessed by individuals without a minimum of 1-10 million dollars of investible assets. People with less money to invest need to go to other investment management providers which sell products instead of objective investment advice. This is not to say that people selling products cannot provide a good rate of return, but I simply must point out that whenever there is a conflict of interest there is always a possibility that one's investment return will be impacted as a direct result. It is also true that selecting an investment advisor charges a fee based on "assets under management" doesn't guarantee exceptional or even good investment returns. It simply means there is no potential conflict of interest and that they should be motivated to grow an investment portfolio.

There are certainly many good investment advisors and investment advisory firms that can help a client create a long term investment strategy. It helps if they are willing to spend the time to listen to the goals and objectives of the investor and keep the investors best interests before their own. This is not always an easy thing to achieve.

It can take concerted efforts by an investor to select his or her investment advisor. You want to make sure the advisor or advisory firm has they appropriate experience, ethics, capability, past performance, and pricing. Many firms provide services to help you conduct the search for the appropriate investment advisor. I recommend that you take the responsibility and the time, effort and commitment as this is an extremely important search in order for you to achieve your long term financial objectives.

Tips for Executing the Plan

Once you have the right advisor and have established your goals and objectives, your advisor will then help you establish an Investment Policy Statement which outlines your goals and objectives. Then it is time for the advisor to execute the plan. The general rule is it's not a good idea to micromanage your surgeon and likewise it's a good idea to give your advisor a respectful level of autonomy. I guess the right word would be to *delegate* the responsibility but never *relegate* your responsibility to your investment advisor. You want to have regular meetings with your advisor to monitor performance and to make sure they are fulfilling the terms of your Investment Policy Statement. It is still your responsibility to monitor your advisor. Again, there are firms that you can retain that are willing to take on this responsibility for you. Individuals with large portfolios typically outsource this service to someone with the capability to monitor this process on an ongoing basis.

As part of your investment policy statement you should also establish a fair and appropriate "measuring stick" or index with which you will measure the performance of your investment portfolio. For example, you might compare on a quarterly basis, investment rates of your equity portfolio with the S&P 500 index or perhaps your bond portfolio with the Lehman Bond index. These indices must be established up front, and then you can determine how well your investment manager is performing. If you are not, then you might need to investigate further to see if the reasons for this are problematic or simply a short term aberration of your investment portfolio. This can only be determined based on the conversation with your investment advisor of why they failed to equal or exceed their benchmark indices. If you are uncomfortable concerning their response then you may need an intermediary to help you monitor your investment advisor.

The Long Term View

Nothing impacts the long term success of your investment performance more than the failure to stick to your investment plan in good times and bad times. Otherwise you will end up chasing your tail and selling investments when you should be buying or moving out of one investment sector when you should be moving in. Many studies have shown that it is very difficult to consistently find the best investments and equally difficult, if not impossible, to time the ups and downs of the investment markets. Therefore, greater performance can be achieved by establishing an appropriate investment strategy and simply sticking to it. It's easy to say this in the beginning but difficult to do when the market is either down or booming. After all, we are all human and we allow non-economic or non-financial information to interfere with our investment strategy. This is typically why investment advisors have much greater results because they have the discipline to "stay the course" for the long term.

This doesn't mean you cannot fire your investment advisor if they fail to execute, but if they don't beat their indices in the first quarter and you decide to terminate and start over again, you might find that you spend a lifetime changing investment managers. Because, just like many of the greatest baseball players in history, they fail to get on base 70% of the time. How long do you stay with the investment advisor when they fail to meet or exceed their benchmark is a difficult question, as it depends on the individual circumstances.

Another key to long term investment performance is a simple concept of compounding. In other words, the longer we can invest our money, the greater the benefits of compounding will impact your long term investment returns. Therefore, putting money in and taking money out does not permit the investment advisor to invest long term. Therefore the money should be set aside for the long term. I might also add that the tax structure favors long term investors as the IRS taxes capital gains at a mere 15% on a security sale held over 12 months and yet the combined federal and state taxes on short term capital gains can be in excess of 45% in some states. Even the taxing authorities are encouraging you to keep your money invested for a longer period.

Telling The Future

People often wonder if investing as we know it today will change in the future. The fact is, people have been asking that question for over 100 years, and even though the world has changed so much, it is funny how basic investment theory has not changed as dramatically. Developing a diversified and balanced investment portfolio still produces the greatest long term results as it did 100 years ago. So although we may invest our money a little differently and there are certainly newer investment programs available to us, nevertheless, the basic principles of investing have remained the same through the years.

Michael Brown, Partner, is a CPA as well as an attorney. He was a Senior Manager with the international accounting firm of KPMG Peat Marwick in Boston before forming Brown & Brown in 1982.

Mike attended the University of Houston and graduated from Holy Cross College. He received his law degree, Cum Laude, from the New England School of Law. Mike speaks regularly on Business and Personal Financial Planning. After many years of serving closely-held businesses and successful individuals, Mike spends much of his time developing strategic plans for the firm's clients, negotiating the purchase and sale of businesses, and working closely with the Brown & Brown staff solving various client financial and strategic issues.

Michael is also actively involved in a number of professional associations such as The Massachusetts Society of CPAs, The American, Massachusetts, and Boston Bar Associations, Small Business Association of New England and the Integrated Advisory Group International, an international association of accounting firms and law firms. Mike serves on the Board of the Community Work Services which is the oldest vocational rehabilitation facility in the country serving multi-handicapped individuals. He is also on the Board of Directors of the Massachusetts Society of CPAs and the Boston Estate Planning Council.

APPENDIX TABLE OF CONTENTS

Appendix A
Brian Grodman

Asset and Liability Summary

ACCT OWNER	ACCT #	03/31/03	06/30/03	09/30/03	12/31/03	03/31/04	06/30/04	9/30/04
Adam's Trust	3GH-106438	$36,000	$41,000	$42,000	$44,000	$45,000	$45,000	$44,000
Jesse's IRA	3GH-050073	$450,000	$491,000	$491,000	$508,000	$519,000	$506,000	$504,000
Talia's Trust	3GH-794811	$889,000	$917,000	$831,000	$893,000	$917,000	$851,000	$848,000
Adam & Jesse	3GH-763055	$227,000	$248,000	$256,000	$270,000	$279,000	$274,000	$268,000
Talia's Indiv Annuity	01-5561262	$100,000	$100,000	$100,000	$100,000	$100,000	$100,000	$100,000
TOTAL		$1,702,000	$1,797,000	$1,720,000	$1,815,000	$1,860,000	$1,776,000	$1,764,000
CASH IN/OUT								
Jesse's IRA	3GH-050073	$0	$0	$0	-$1,930	$0	$0	$0
Adam & Jesse	3GH-763055	$0	-$4,680	-$100,000	-$4,264	-$2,140	-$55,144	$0
Talia's Trust	3GH-794811	$0	$0	$0	$0	$0	-$7,650	-$1,250

Appendix B
William Barton Boyer, Parsec Financial

Do You Want to Be Independently Wealthy?

<u>Assumptions</u>

1. Save 15% of your pre-tax income for 36 years.
2. Do as much as possible in tax favored accounts such as Roth IRAs and 401K/Profit Sharing Plans.
3. This is based on a beginning $30,000 income, rising 4% per year. Adjust your situation, up or down, from the $30,000 example.
4. Total stock market results, estimated 10% annually in the future (10.2% annually for large company, 12.1% for small company from 1925-2002).
5. Begin spending at 5% annually in retirement. Carefully study the 5-10% retirement spending examples.

Year	Income	15% Savings	Portfolio
1	$30,000	$4,500	$4,706
5	35,096	5,264	30,811
9	41,057	6,158	73,188
13	48,031	7,205	131,087
17	56,190	8,429	230,351
21	65,735	9,860	382,210
25	76,901	11,536	612,186
30	93,562	14,034	1,068,283
36	118,385	17,758	2,021,305
	-17,758	-------	x 5%
	$100,627		$101,065

Save 20% annually: Have 33.3% more!

Save 7.5% annually: Have 50% less!

Allocate 50% equities/50% fixed income; expect 50% less money!

YOU decide your own future; you are the Chairman and CEO of You, Inc.! Choose to be successful.

Appendix C
William Barton Boyer, Parsec Financial

WHO IS THE LOSER?

	Treasury Bills Retiree 1 - Spend All Income		S&P 500 Retiree 2 - Spend 5% - 10%	
12-31-64	$1,000,000	$39,300	$1,000,000	$50,000
12-31-69	$1,000,000	$65,200	$979,485	$56,618
12-31-74	$1,000,000	$58,000	$649,266	$59,230
12-31-79	$1,000,000	$112,400	$932,874	$59,230
12-31-84	$1,000,000	$77,200	$1,459,768	$72,070
12-31-89	$1,000,000	$78,100	$2,985,623	$118,018
12-31-94	$1,000,000	$56,000	$3,560,881	$184,866
12-31-99	$1,000,000	$60,300	$10,233,880	$440,963
12-31-02	$1,000,000	$11,900	$5,116,317	$511,631
12-31-03	$1,000,000	$9,100	$6,072,557	$511,631
Total Spending		$2,367,900		$6,543,624
Total Spending & Principal		$3,367,900		$12,616,181
Total Spending		$2,367,900		$6,543,624

*Statistical Source: Ibbotson Associates

Appendix D
William Barton Boyer, Parsec Financial

ANNUAL SPENDING FROM A 100% EQUITY S&P 500 PORTFOLIO.
SPEND 5% WHENEVER 5% IS A HIGHER SPENDING LEVEL.
LEVEL SPENDING WHEN ABOVE 5% (NOT TO EXCEED 10%).
THE GOAL - STABLE OR RISING SPENDING.

Value	Principal	5-10% Spending of The Previous Year's
12-31-64	$1,000,000	
12-31-65	$1,074,500	$50,000
12-31-66	$912,680	$53,725
12-31-67	$1,077,816	$53,725
12-31-68	$1,132,353	$53,890
12-31-69	$979,485	$56,618
12-31-70	$962,144	$56,618
12-31-71	$1,043,209	$56,618
12-31-72	$1,184,592	$56,618
12-31-73	$963,547	$59,230
12-31-74	$649,266	$59,230
12-31-75	$831,563	$59,230
12-31-76	$970,578	$59,230
12-31-77	$841,660	$59,230
12-31-78	$837,643	$59,230
12-31-79	$932,874	$59,230
12-31-80	$1,176,081	$59,230
12-31-81	$1,059,105	$59,230
12-31-82	$1,226,629	$59,230
12-31-83	$1,441,412	$61,331
12-31-84	$1,459,768	$72,070
12-31-85	$1,856,177	$72,986
12-31-86	$2,106,204	$92,809
12-31-87	$2,111,048	$105,310
12-31-88	$2,360,363	$105,552
12-31-89	$2,985,623	$118,018
12-31-90	$2,741,697	$149,281

12-31-91	$3,430,004	$149,281
12-31-92	$3,521,585	$171,500
12-31-93	$3,697,712	$176,079
12-31-94	$3,560,881	$184,866
12-31-95	$4,708,853	$184,866
12-31-96	$5,559,743	$235,443
12-31-97	$7,136,486	$277,987
12-31-98	$8,819,269	$356,824
12-31-99	$10,233,880	$440,963
12-31-00	$8,789,879	$511,694
12-31-01	$7,233,947	$511,694
12-31-02	$5,116,317	$511,694
12-31-03	$6,072,557	$511,632
Year 2004 Spending		$511,632

TOTAL SPENDING (SO FAR) **$6,543,624**

*Statistical Source: Ibbotson Associates

Appendix E
William Barton Boyer, Parsec Financial

ANNUAL SPENDING FROM A 100% EQUITY S&P 500 PORTFOLIO.
SPEND 5% WHENEVER 5% IS A HIGHER SPENDING LEVEL.
LEVEL SPENDING WHEN ABOVE 5% (NOT TO EXCEED 10%).
THE GOAL - STABLE OR RISING SPENDING.

Spending	Principal	5-10%
12-31-74	$1,000,000	
12-31-75	$1,322,000	$50,000
12-31-76	$1,571,065	$66,100
12-31-77	$1,379,709	$78,553
12-31-78	$1,391,665	$78,553
12-31-79	$1,569,735	$78,553
12-31-80	$2,000,090	$78,553
12-31-81	$1,801,881	$100,004
12-31-82	$2,087,660	$100,004
12-31-83	$2,453,209	$104,383
12-31-84	$2,484,365	$122,660
12-31-85	$3,159,119	$124,218
12-31-86	$3,584,652	$157,956
12-31-87	$3,592,897	$179,233
12-31-88	$4,017,218	$179,645
12-31-89	$5,081,379	$200,861
12-31-90	$4,666,320	$254,069
12-31-91	$5,832,564	$254,069
12-31-92	$5,988,293	$291,628
12-31-93	$6,287,109	$299,415
12-31-94	$6,079,006	$314,355
12-31-95	$8,040,023	$314,355
12-31-96	$9,492,855	$402,001
12-31-97	$12,185,029	$474,643
12-31-98	$15,058,258	$609,251
12-31-99	$17,473,602	$752,913
12-31-00	$15,008,077	$873,680
12-31-01	$12,351,437	$873,680

12-31-02	$8,735,738	$873,680
12-31-03	$10,368,447	$873,574
Year 2004 Spending		$873,574

TOTAL SPENDING (SO FAR)	**$10,034,163**

*Statistical Source: Ibbotson Associates

Appendix F
William Barton Boyer, Parsec Financial

Dollar Cost Averaging
Buying and Spending
S&P 500 Portfolio

Assumptions

1. Buy January 1, 1929, and every January 1 thereafter for thirty years, reinvest income for eleven more years. Begin buying at the worst possible time. Suffer ALL the declines along the way.
2. Annual savings begins with $1,000, increasing 5% annually, save for thirty years.
3. Begin spending 5-10% annually from the portfolio beginning the 41st year. Begin spending just prior to the worst financial decade in the last sixty years.

YEAR	SAVE	CUMULATIVE SAVINGS	5-10% ANNUAL PORTFOLIO*	SPENDING
1929	$ 1,000	$ 1,000	$ 915	
1930	1,050	2,050	1,476	
1931	1,102	3,152	1,461	
1932	1,157	4,309	2,406	
1933	1,215	5,524	5,576	
1938	1,551	12,575	18,531	
1943	1,980	21,576	34,376	
1948	2,527	33,064	71,820	
1953	3,225	47,724	185,736	
1958	4,116	66,434	539,938	
1963			863,768	
1969			1,282,009	
1970	Review Historical 5-10% Spending			$64,100

* Statistical source: Ibbotson Associates

Appendix G
William Barton Boyer, Parsec Financial

Alternative Retirement Spending Option,
Eliminate Stock Market Volatility

Assumptions

1. Buy a fixed annuity from a large, well respected insurance company.
2. Ages 65 and 65, joint and survivor annuity.
3. Twenty years certain payments.

	Principal	Payment
12-31-01	$1,000,000	
2003	☹	$59,700
2008	☹	$59,700
2013	☹	$59,700
2018	☹	$59,700
2023	☹	$59,700
2028	☹	$59,700
2030	☹	$59,700
Total	☹	$1,611,900

(Sorry Kids!)

CEO Best Practices

Management & Leadership Strategies From 200+ C-Level Executives

This insider look at succeeding as a top executive is written by C-Level professionals (CEOs, CFOs, CTOs, CMOs) from the world's leading companies. Each executive shares their knowledge on how to get an edge in business, from leading a company to making money in a down economy to increasing your efficiencies in all areas of your business (marketing, financial, technology, hr, and more). Also covered are over 250 specific, proven innovative strategies and methodologies practiced by leading executives and CEOs that have helped them gain an edge. This report is designed to give you insight into the leading executives of the world, and assist you in developing additional ideas in all areas of your business that can help you be even more successful as a top executive.

WRITTEN BY C-LEVEL EXECUTIVES FROM COMPANIES AT:

Advanced Fibre Communications, American Express, American Standard Companies, AmeriVest Properties, AT Kearney, AT&T Wireless, Bank of America, Barclays, BDO Seidman, BearingPoint (Formerly KPMG Consulting), BEA Systems, Best Buy, BMC Software, Boeing, Booz-Allen Hamilton, Corning, Countrywide, Credit Suisse First Boston, Deutsche Bank, Drake Beam Morin, Duke Energy, Ernst & Young, FedEx, First Consulting Group, Ford Motor Co., Frost & Sullivan, General Electric, IBM, Interpublic Group, KPMG, LandAmerica, Mack-Cali Realty Corporation, Merrill Lynch, Micron Technology, Milliman & Robertson, Novell, Office Depot, On Semiconductor, Oxford Health, PeopleSoft, Perot Systems, Prudential, Salomon Smith Barney, Staples, Tellabs, The Coca-Cola Company, Unilever, Verizon, VoiceStream Wireless, Webster Financial Corporation, Weil, Gotshal & Manges, Yahoo!

$219.95

Call 1-866-Aspatore (277-2867) to Order Today!

Other Best Sellers

- Ninety-Six and Too Busy to Die - Life Beyond the Age of Dying - $24.95
- Technology Blueprints - Strategies for Optimizing and Aligning Technology Strategy & Business - $69.95
- The CEO's Guide to Information Availability - Why Keeping People & Information Connected is Every Leader's New Priority - $27.95
- Being There Without Going There - Managing Teams Across Time Zones, Locations and Corporate Boundaries - $24.95
- Profitable Customer Relationships - CEOs from Leading Software Companies on using Technology to Maxmize Acquisition, Retention & Loyalty - $27.95
- The Entrepreneurial Problem Solver - Leading CEOs on How to Think Like an Entrepreneur and Solve Any Problem for Your Team/Company - $27.95
- The Philanthropic Executive - Establishing a Charitable Plan for Individuals & Businesses - $27.95
- The Golf Course Locator for Business Professionals - Organized by Closest to Largest 500 Companies, Cities & Airports - $12.95
- Living Longer Working Stronger - 7 Steps to Capitalizing on Better Health - $14.95
- Business Travel Bible - Must Have Phone Numbers, Business Resources, Maps & Emergency Info - $19.95
- ExecRecs - Executive Recommendations for the Best Business Products & Services Professionals Use to Excel - $14.95

Call 1-866-Aspatore (277-2867) to Order

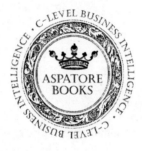